Hispanic/Latino Adult Tobacco Survey Guidance Document

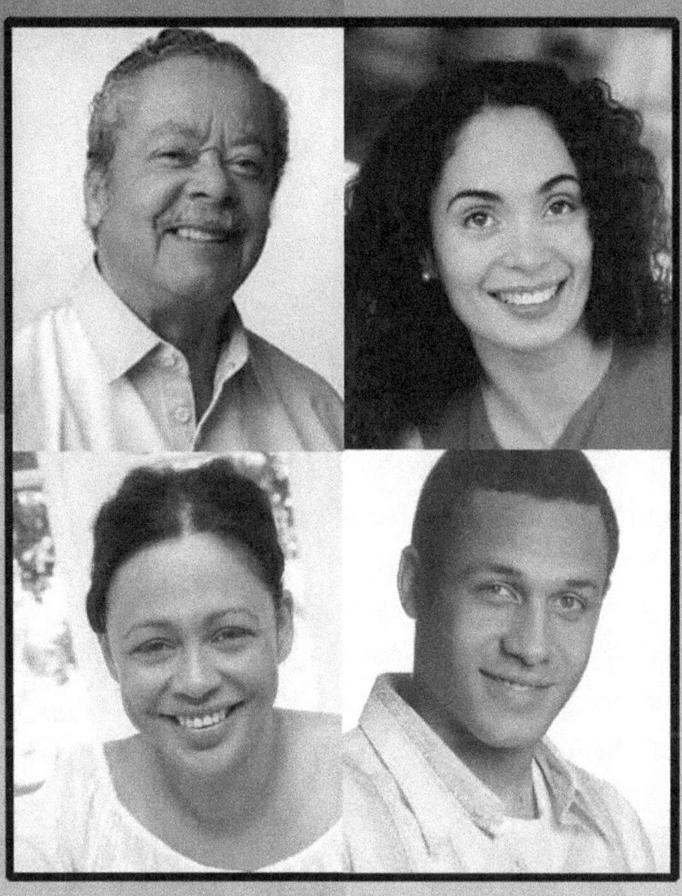

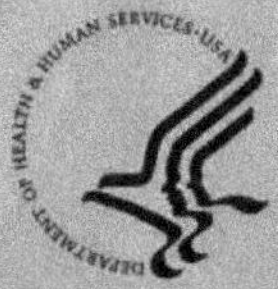

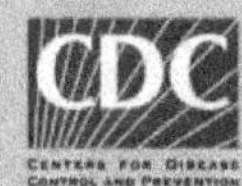

Contents

Section **Page**

A. Introduction **1**

B. Instruments **2**

B.1 Comparison of H/L ATS Smoking Status Variables with Those on the General Population State ATS 2

B.2 Core Module Q-by-Qs 3

B.2.1 Section 1: General Health 4

B.2.2 Section 2: Cigarette Smoking 4

B.2.3 Section 3: Cessation 5

B.2.4 Section 4: Secondhand Smoke 7

B.2.5 Section 5: Risk Perception and Social Influences 8

B.2.6 Section 6: Demographic Items 9

B.3 Optional Modules Q-by-Qs 11

B.3.1 Section A: Detailed Demographic Items 11

B.3.2 Section B: Detailed Tobacco Use Questions 12

B.3.3 Section C: Detailed Cessation Questions 12

B.3.4 Section D: Detailed Environmental Tobacco Smoke Questions 12

B.3.5 Section E: Health and Social Influences 13

B.3.6 Section F: Policy Issues 13

B.3.7 Section G: Parental Involvement 13

B.3.8 Section H: Media Exposure 14

B.4 Screeners 14

B.5 Advance Letters 15

B.6 Informed Consent Text and Forms 16

C. Sampling and Weighting **18**

C.1 Sampling in Three Case Study Surveys 18

C.1.1 New York, New York: Telephone Survey in Urban Area with Moderate Concentration of Hispanic and Latino Persons 19

C.1.2 Miami, Florida: Telephone Survey in Urban Area with Higher Concentration of Hispanic and Latino Persons 21

C.1.3 El Paso, Texas: In-person Survey in Border Areas with High Concentration of Hispanic and Latino Persons 22

C.2 Within-household Sampling 24
C.2.1 Reducing Gender Bias in Respondent Selection 25
C.2.2 Respondent Selection in Multifamily Hispanic Households. 25
C.2.3 Additional Considerations 26
C.3 Weighting Methods in the Three H/L ATS Case studies 26
C.3.1 Sample Weights 27
C.3.2 Weight Calculation 27
C.3.3 Lack of Known Totals to Calibrate Weights 28
C.3.4 Statistical Software for Complex Survey Designs 29

D. Analysis and Reporting **30**

D.1 Tobacco Use Among Young Adults 30
D.1.1 Example 1: Current Smoking Levels 31
D.1.2 Example 2: Age at Initiation of Smoking 33
D.2 Exposure to Secondhand Smoke 34
D.2.1 Example 1: Exposure to Secondhand Smoke at Home 34
D.2.2 Example 2: Exposure of Nonsmokers to Workplace Secondhand Smoke 36
D.2.3 Example 3: Attitudes Toward Laws on Clean Indoor Air 37
D.3 Smoking Cessation 38
D.3.1 Example 1: Stages of Change 38
D.3.2 Example 2: Methods Used to Quit at Last Quit Attempt 39
D.3.3 Example 3: Length of Abstinence Among Former Smokers 39
D.4 Use of Additional Data Sets 40
D.4.1 Example 1: Occupational Differences in Workplace Smoking Policies 40
D.4.2 Example 2: Merging H/L ATS Data with Environmental Data 41

E. Enhancing Response Rates **43**

F. Background, References, and Resources **45**

F.1 Background to the Development of the H/L ATS 45
F.1.1 Purpose of a Culturally Appropriate H/L ATS 45
F.1.2 Design of the H/L ATS Questionnaires and Survey Methodology 47
F.1.3 Development of Spanish Versions of the H/L ATS 48
F.2 References and Resources 50
F.2.1 Background to Hispanic/Latino Surveying and the ATS 50
F.2.2 Instrumentation 51
F.2.3 Sampling and Weighting 53

F.2.4 Analysis and Reporting 55
F.2.5 Enhancing Response Rates 56
F.3 Contacts 56

Appendices

A: Advance Letter to Potential Households, Telephone Survey (English) A-1
B: Advance Letter to Potential Households, Telephone Survey (Spanish) B-1
C: Advance Letter to Potential Households, In-person Survey (English) C-1
D: Advance Letter to Potential Households, In-person Survey (Spanish) D-1
E: Informed Consent Form, In-person Survey (English) E-1
F: Informed Consent Form, In-person Survey (Spanish) F-1
G: Informed Consent Text, Telephone Survey (English) G-1
H: Informed Consent Text, Telephone Survey (Spanish) H-1

Tables

Number **Page**

C-1 Description of the Three H/L ATS Case Study Sites 19
D-1 H/L ATS Questions Addressed in Tables D-2 Through D-7 31
D-2 "Current," "Former," and "Never" Smokers Among All Hispanic Persons Aged 18 to 24, by Country of Birth (Percentage) 31
D-3 Number of Cigarettes Smoked Daily by "Every Day" and "Some Days" Hispanic Smokers Aged 18 to 24, by Country of Birth (Percentage) 32
D-4 Whether Hispanic Adults Aged 18 to 24 Smoked 100 Cigarettes in Their Lifetime, by Age (Percentage) 32
D-5 "Current," "Former," and "Never Smokers" Among All Hispanic Persons Aged 18 to 19, by Respondent's Age Upon First Entry into the United States (Percentage) 33
D-6 Age at Which Hispanic Persons Aged 30 or Older First Smoked a Cigarette, by Education (Percentage) 33
D-7 Use of Menthol Cigarettes Among Hispanic Smokers Aged 18 to 24, by Perceived Benefits of Quitting (Percentage) 34
D-8 H/L ATS Questions Addressed in Tables D-9 Through D-13 34
D-9 Home Smoking Rules Among All Hispanic Adults, by Income (Percentage) 35
D-10 Number of Days in Last Week That Someone Smoked Inside Home, by Language Generally Spoken by Adult Respondent (Percentage) 35
D-11 Number of Smokers in Home, by Age of Children in Home (Percentage) 36
D-12 Workplace Smoking Policy for Indoor Work Areas and Indoor Public Areas Used by Hispanic Nonsmoking Workers, by Education (Percentage) 37
D-13 Whether Hispanic Adult Respondents Think Smoking Should Be Prohibited in Worksites and Other Indoor Places, by Smoking Status (Percentage) 38
D-14 H/L ATS Questions Addressed in Tables D-15 Through D-17 38
D-15 Hispanic Current Smokers' Stage of Change Toward Smoking Cessation, by Whether Spouse or Partner Uses Tobacco (Percentage) 39
D-16 Methods Used to Quit Smoking Among Hispanic Current and Former Smokers, by Gender (Percentage) 39
D-17 Length of Abstinence Among Hispanic Current and Former Smokers, by Age (Percentage) 40
D-18 H/L ATS Questions Addressed in Tables D-19 and D-20 40
D-19 U.S. Employed Smokers Who Work in Smoke-free, Smoking-allowed, and No-policy Workplaces, by Occupation (Percentage) 41
D-20 Beliefs About the Harmful Effects of Breathing Secondhand Smoke, by Strength of Local Clean Indoor Air Laws (Percentage) 41
F-1 National Origin, City of Residence, and Language of Interview for Respondents to the H/L ATS Cognitive Testing 50

A. INTRODUCTION

The Hispanic/Latino Adult Tobacco Survey (H/L ATS) is designed to measure the tobacco-related behaviors, knowledge, attitudes, and opinions of Hispanic and Latino persons. While the H/L ATS is based on the General Population State ATS and will generate comparable results, it is uniquely suited for administration among Hispanic/Latino populations: the questions asked and vocabulary used reflect the experience and language of Hispanic/Latino persons. In addition, the Spanish translation was carefully developed to be understood by Spanish-speakers from various countries of origin.

To facilitate comparisons, a symbol appears next to each H/L ATS module question to indicate how that question compares with its counterpart on the General Population State ATS: identical (▲), very similar but not identical (◆), or similar but not identical (■). The symbol for "very similar but not identical" may mean, for example, that the same wording appears in both question versions but in a different order; whereas the symbol for "similar but not identical" may mean the two versions differ in wording. New questions not originally included on the General Population State ATS are indicated (●).

This guide highlights what is unique to the H/L ATS, as opposed to the General Population State ATS, and provides tips for meeting the unique challenges of conducting a population-based sample survey among the Hispanic/Latino population.

The guide is organized into five main sections:

- Instruments
- Sampling and Weighting
- Analysis and Reporting
- Enhancing Response Rates
- Background, References, and Resources

For more information and background on the General Population State ATS, see *Guidelines for Conducting General Population State Adult Tobacco Surveys* (Mariolis, in press).

This guide was developed by the Centers for Disease Control and Prevention's (CDC) Office on Smoking and Health (OSH). For additional information, contact this office by e-mail at tobaccoinfo@cdc.gov or by phone at 1-800-CDC-INFO. Visit the OSH Online Publications Catalog to order OSH publications and materials.

The H/L ATS instruments and survey materials were approved by the Office of Management and Budget (OMB) for use by CDC in New York, Florida, and Texas. This approval does not extend to other uses of the H/L ATS. Use in other locations, by CDC or any other researcher, requires approval from pertinent authorities. It may be helpful when applying for such approval to reference the approval provided by OMB to CDC.

B. INSTRUMENTS

The Hispanic/Latino Adult Tobacco Survey (H/L ATS) consists of six core and eight optional modules. The core constitutes the basic set of questions that must be asked for the study. Optional questions can be selectively added, depending on local interest, time, and cost considerations. Survey question by survey question, this section provides users specific survey-administration guidance based on cognitive testing; in addition, it explains the purpose and correct use of the H/L ATS Screener, advance letters, and informed consent materials.

B.1 Comparison of H/L ATS Smoking Status Variables with Those on the General Population State ATS

The smoking status of respondents (Rs) determines the path they follow through the questionnaire. Respondents can be either current smokers or former smokers, or they may have never been smokers in their lives, according to the working definitions in the survey. This same classification of Rs by smoking status is used in the General Population State ATS.

Symbols indicate how H/L ATS questions compare with their counterparts on the General Population State ATS: ▲ identical; ◆ very similar; ■ similar; ● new.

Responses to two key questions classify Rs' smoking status:

■ **Q4:** In your entire life, have you smoked at least 100 cigarettes, about five packs? Responses: "Yes," "No," "Don't know/Not sure," or "Refused."

◆ **Q5:** Do you now smoke cigarettes every day, some days, or not at all? Responses: "Every day," "Some days," "Not at all," "Don't know/Not sure," or "Refused."

Current smokers. A current smoker is an R who has smoked at least 100 cigarettes in his lifetime and was smoking every day or some days at the time of survey. The R will have answered "Yes" to Q4, and "Every day" or "Some days" to Q5.

Former smokers. A former smoker is an R who has smoked at least 100 cigarettes during his lifetime and currently does not smoke. The R will have answered "Yes" to Q4, and "Not at all" to Q5.

Never smokers. The R is classified as never having smoked if he says he has not smoked at least 100 cigarettes during his lifetime. The R will have answered "No" to Q4, and "Not at all" to Q5.

Although Q6 is not used to determine smoking status, it can be used to better distinguish the occasional smoker from other types of smokers:

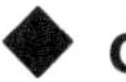 **Q6:** During the past 30 days, on how many days did you smoke cigarettes? Responses: "None," Number of Days ("1" to "30"), "Don't know/Not sure," or "Refused."

Occasional smokers are more common in Hispanic/Latino populations, so this category of smokers is of greater interest to public health practitioners in Hispanic/Latino communities.

B.2 Core Module Q-by-Qs

The question-by-question specifications (Q-by-Qs) in this section complement and augment materials prepared for the General Population State ATS. The core module of the H/L ATS covers six topics:

1. General Health
2. Cigarette Smoking
3. Cessation
4. Secondhand Smoke
5. Risk Perception and Social Influences
6. Demographic Items

The core module should be administered in full to obtain the information required to determine smoking status and its correlates. The optional modules can be used selectively, depending on the specific research or evaluation objectives and the availability of funds to design and conduct a longer interview.

With the exception of Cessation, all sections have at least some questions for all kinds of Rs. Cessation questions are asked of both current and former smokers, but not of those Rs who, according to the H/L ATS definition, have never smoked.

Included below are Q-by-Qs for the core module. These Q-by-Qs focus on issues uncovered through cognitive testing of the H/L ATS with approximately 60 Hispanic/Latino persons (about three fourths of whom were tested in Spanish and one fourth in English). The testing was conducted to ascertain how the H/L ATS questions are interpreted and understood by Hispanic/Latino persons. The results of the testing as presented in these Q-by-Qs highlight the following:

- Words and terms that seemed to be confusing or required clarification.
- Ways to probe ambiguous responses.
- Suggestions on how to capture meaningful and consistent responses.

The Optional Modules Q-by-Qs appear in Section B.3.

Because the text of each question is not included in these Q-by-Qs, users of the guide may want to have a printout of the H/L ATS on hand:

- H/L ATS Core Module (in English)
- H/L ATS Core Module (Spanish, with English Instructions for Programmers and Interviewers)
- H/L ATS Preguntas principales (totalmente en español)

B.2.1 Section 1: General Health

The General Health section (Q1) consists of a single question asking R to give his subjective evaluation of his general health.

 **Q1:** ***General health status.*** In the cognitive interviews, Rs generally avoided selecting the top two response options for this question. Rs who felt physically well but had been some time without a physician's examination were reluctant to choose these responses, because they could not be sure nothing was wrong with their health. The same was true for those who felt very well but knew they had not followed a healthy lifestyle (e.g., smokers or those who did not exercise).

B.2.2 Section 2: Cigarette Smoking

The nine questions about cigarette smoking (Q2 to Q10) elicit information about the R's lifetime and current cigarette smoking. Q4 and Q5 are used to determine the smoking status of an R. Determining smoking status is critical because it dictates the path the R will take through the instrument (see Section B.2).

Rs are asked if they have ever smoked a cigarette in their lifetime and, if so, at what age they first smoked. Rs who have smoked are asked if they have smoked at least 100 cigarettes in their lives. Rs who report smoking in the past 30 days are asked how many days they have smoked in the past 30, how many cigarettes they have smoked per day, how soon they first smoke after waking up, what their most frequently smoked brand is, and whether they smoke menthol cigarettes.

 **Q2:** ***Whether R has ever smoked a cigarette.*** This question asks the R if he has ever smoked a cigarette, even one or two puffs. The reference period is the R's entire life. As with the General Population State ATS, all questions regarding cigarette smoking are about tobacco cigarettes only and do not include marijuana or any other smoked substances rolled in paper.

The Spanish translation of the English word *puffs* presents issues. Rs of different national origins refer to *puffs* with different Spanish words. Terms tested in cognitive interviews (*pitadas* and *jaladas*) were not universally understood; therefore, the term was changed to *probadas* (literally, *tries*) for the Spanish versions of the H/L ATS.

Cigarettes are customarily called *cigarros* by Mexican-origin Rs and are called *cigarrillos* by most other Spanish-speakers. *Cigarro* cannot be used for this question, because it means *cigar* for natives of several countries. Testing indicated, however, that even those Rs who use *cigarro* for *cigarette* understand *cigarrillo* as *cigarette*.

◆ **Q3:** ***Age at R's first time smoking.*** This question is asked only of those who answered "Yes" in Q2. Responses must be in years of age. Responses such as "5 years ago" or "in my last year of high school" should be probed for exact age.

■ **Q4:** ***Whether R has smoked at least 100 cigarettes in his lifetime.*** This question is intended to elicit whether the R has smoked a total of 100 cigarettes in his lifetime, not in a single day. In testing it appeared that smokers are accustomed to reporting daily cigarette consumption and tend to hear this question as asking about a single day. The interviewer should stress "not on a single day." Training should focus on this issue because this question is key to determining Rs' smoking status. As applies to any question, if an R says something that suggests he has misunderstood the question, the interviewer should repeat the question or that part of it that has been misunderstood.

◆ **Q5:** ***Whether R currently smokes every day, some days, or not at all.*** The reference period for this question is the present, without further definition. This question elicits current smoking status and is used to identify the category of "current smokers."

◆ **Q6:** ***Days R smoked in the past 30.*** The reference period is the 30 days before the interview date. Responses not provided in number of days (responses given as frequency—e.g., "every day" or "twice a week") should be probed, with stress on "how many days."

▲ **Q7:** ***Cigarettes smoked per day on days when R smoked in the past 30.*** The reference period is the 30 days before the interview date. The question is intended to elicit average daily consumption on days when R smoked. In cognitive testing, some Rs answered in ways that may pose calculation problems for the interviewers. Interviewers should practice probing or coding answers such as "I smoke a pack in 3 days" or "I smoke two packs in a day and a half."

▲ **Q8:** ***How soon after waking R smokes the first cigarette.*** This question offers categories to elicit the time elapsed between R's waking and the first cigarette smoking of the day. The question indicates that the response options must be read aloud to the R. Some Rs associate smoking with specific activities and may first answer in that way (e.g., "I light up right after breakfast"). Such uncodable responses should be probed; the response categories, repeated.

▲ **Q9:** ***Brand R most frequently smokes.*** The list of cigarette brands offered includes generic (or no-brand) cigarettes.

▲ **Q10:** ***Whether R smokes menthols.*** The question aims to elicit whether R usually smokes menthol cigarettes.

B.2.3 Section 3: Cessation

The Cessation section consists of 11 questions (Q11 to Q21) that elicit information on the following subjects: attempts to quit smoking (Q11 and Q12), methods of quitting (Q13 and

Q14), stages of change for quitting (Q15 and Q16), physician and health professionals' advice (Q17 to Q20), and nontraditional methods of quitting (Q21). These questions are asked of "current smokers." Selected items are also asked of "former smokers" who quit in the previous 5 years.

▲ **Q11:** ***How long since last cigarette.*** It is important to read the response categories for this question to R. In cognitive testing, when response options were not explicitly offered, Rs gave complex answers that would be difficult for interviewers to code. Time references given in parentheses are for interviewers to use at their discretion, to aid processing of R's answer or to probe an unclear response.

▲ **Q12:** ***Quit attempts lasting longer than 1 day.*** It is important to ensure that R listens to this entire question before answering; otherwise, he may answer "Yes" for reasons other than quitting smoking for a day or longer (e.g., if he was in the hospital for a day or longer).

▲ **Q13:** ***Use of nicotine or other medications to help quit.*** This question is asked only of "current smokers" who made a quit attempt in the past year or of "former smokers" who quit in the past 5 years. Alternate introductions are provided for each of these two types of R.

▲ **Q14:** ***Use of classes or counseling to help quit.*** This question is asked only of "current smokers" who made a quit attempt in the past year or of "former smokers" who quit in the past 5 years. Alternate introductions are provided for each of these two types of R.

▲ **Q15:** ***Considering quitting within the next 6 months.*** This question is asked only of "current smokers."

■ **Q16:** ***When planning to quit.*** This question is asked only of "current smokers" who are seriously considering stopping smoking within the next 6 months. Rs that do not have specific plans to quit at a certain time should be coded as "Don't know/Not sure."

▲ **Q17:** ***Health checkup or received care in the past 12 months.*** Both "current smokers" and "former smokers" who quit in the past 5 years answer this item.

▲ **Q18:** ***Health professional advised R not to smoke.*** This and subsequent items in this section are asked only of Rs who answered "Yes" at Q17.

▲ **Q19:** ***Health professional asked R if he smokes.*** This question is asked only of Rs who were *not* advised by a health professional to quit smoking ("No" at Q18).

▲ **Q20a–d:** ***Health professional recommended quit aids.*** This sequence is asked of any R whose health care professional either advised against smoking or asked R whether he smoked.

B.2.4 Section 4: Secondhand Smoke

The Secondhand Smoke section contains 15 questions (Q22 to Q34). They establish R's secondhand smoke exposure outside work (Q22 to Q25), workplace secondhand smoke policy and exposure (Q26 to Q33), and attitudes about rules on clean indoor air (Q34).

● **Q22:** ***Number of adults living in R's household.*** This may be a sensitive question for Rs who live in multifamily households, which sometimes violate maximum-occupancy rules. If R's answer indicates that he is counting only his own relatives, the interviewer should state that the question is about all adults in the household, whether or not they are related to R.

A few cognitive-interview Rs who were recent immigrants interpreted *su hogar* (in English, "your household") as referring to their household in their country of origin. The intent of this question is to ask about R's current household in the United States, no matter how temporary that may feel to R.

◆ **Q23:** ***Number of adult household members who smoke.*** This question is about only tobacco smoking.

■ **Q24:** ***Smoking of tobacco inside the home.*** The interviewer should stress the word *inside* to make sure Rs are not including outdoor locations of the home. In cognitive testing, some Rs were including outdoor locations, such as yards.

■ **Q25:** ***Rules about smoking inside R's home.*** If an R provides an answer that is not one of those listed, the interviewer should reread the categories and ask the R to select from among the responses provided. Responses such as "You can smoke only outside" or "We allow smoking only out in the yard" should be probed, with stress on the word *inside.*

■ **Q26:** ***R's working status.*** This question elicits R's working status as part of the general information about R and in order to determine whether he should be asked the subsequent questions about smoking in the workplace. Interviewers should read each category slowly and give R the opportunity to process each response option, but interviewers should read all response options before accepting one as an answer.

▲ **Q27:** ***R's work location—indoors or not.*** This question is asked to determine whether R should be asked about indoor smoking at work.

▲ **Q28:** ***Smoking in R's work area.*** No definition is provided for *work area.* It is whatever R defines as his work area. Work areas can vary widely. A traveling salesman may consider a car as his work area. Other examples of *work area* are cubicle, jobsite, and warehouse.

● **Q29:** ***Official policy about smoking at work.*** This yes/no question often elicits descriptions of the policy that will be elicited in the two subsequent questions. Interviewers should be prepared to say something such as "The next question asks what the policy is."

◆ **Q30:** ***Official smoking policy for work areas.*** This question often elicits answers such as "We can smoke only outside." The question should then be repeated, with stress on the term *work areas.*

◆ **Q31:** ***Official smoking policy for indoor public areas.*** Lobbies, restrooms, and lunchrooms are offered to the R as examples only. Not all jobs have lobbies or lunchrooms. Some jobs have only common areas, such as restrooms or hallways.

◆ **Q32:** ***Attitude about prohibition of smoking in indoor work areas.*** In cognitive testing, some Rs answered without selecting one of the response options, saying, for example, "It should be allowed in some areas" or "There should be a smoking area." The interviewer should repeat the response options so that R selects one.

▲ **Q33:** ***Exposure to smoke in car.*** The interviewer should be sure R understands that "someone smoking" does not refer to R himself: the person smoking must be someone else.

● **Q34a–e:** ***Attitude about prohibition of smoking in public places.*** In cognitive testing, some Rs answered without selecting one of the response options, saying, for example, "It should be allowed in some areas" or "There should be a smoking area." The interviewer should repeat the response options so that R selects one.

The clarifications in parentheses in Q34a and Q34b should be read in all instances.

B.2.5 Section 5: Risk Perception and Social Influences

The Risk Perception and Social Influences section consists of six questions (Q35 to Q40) that together cover R's perception of risk from smoking (Q35) and from secondhand smoke (Q36 to Q39), as well as R's views about prohibiting smoking in specific indoor places (Q40). All questions are asked of all Rs.

▲ **Q36:** ***Perceived harm in breathing smoke from others' cigarettes.*** Many cognitive-interview Rs felt that breathing smoke from the cigarettes of others was as bad as, if not worse than, smoking itself.

● **Q37a–f:** ***Health effects from secondhand smoke.*** The stem of this question is repeated every two items to continually remind R that the question is about *secondhand smoke* (not about smoking).

In Q37c and Q37e, if R is not familiar with colon cancer or with crib death, code answer as "Don't know" (code 7).

● **Q38:** ***Health danger of regular exposure to secondhand smoke.*** Rs may have different motivations for selecting a response. Some may be without health worries because they do not believe exposure to secondhand smoke is harmful, but others may give the same answer only because they are already smokers themselves. Whatever R's motivation, his response choice is what matters.

● **Q39:** ***Secondhand smoke as a health hazard or annoyance.*** It is important that R hear all responses before selecting one.

B.2.6 Section 6: Demographic Items

The Demographic Items section contains 16 questions (Q41 to Q56) that elicit basic demographic information on R. They cover R's age, gender, education, country of birth (and, for immigrants, age at immigration and total number of years lived in the United States), marital status, sexual identification, number of children in the household by age, use of English and Spanish, and household income. Additional questions ask about use of tobacco by R's current spouse or partner, zip code, and medical coverage status. At the end of the section, which is also the end of the core sections, the interviewer is asked to enter the date of interview and code whether the interview was conducted in English or in Spanish.

◆ **Q41:** ***Age.*** Rs occasionally may prefer not to disclose their age. The interviewer should reassure R that responses to the survey are securely protected, and then the interviewer should repeat the question.

● **Q42:** ***Gender.*** When certain of the answer, the interviewer may code gender without asking R for it. Whenever uncertain, though, the interviewer must ask. To make asking less awkward, the interviewer may preface the question by saying, "I'm required to ask this."

▲ **Q43:** ***Marital status.*** This question may elicit multiple answers. For example, a person may be both separated and living with someone other than his spouse, or be still married but separated. If the R offers multiple responses, all responses should be recorded.

● **Q44:** ***Children.*** Respondents may be wary of disclosing the age of children in the home. In such cases, the interviewer should reassure R that all answers are confidential.

● **Q45:** ***Country of birth.*** Any response that does not appear on the list of countries should be entered under "Other."

● **Q46:** ***Age at immigration.*** This question elicits the age at which R first moved to the United States. For those who came and left, R's age at *first* date of immigration should be recorded here.

Some Rs will answer by providing the year of immigration. If so, the interviewer should skip the boxes for entering age and enter the year in the boxes provided below the age response boxes.

● **Q47–48:** ***Spanish/English use by R.*** For these two questions, the order of response options in the Spanish versions is the reverse of those in the English version, but they have the same corresponding codes. That is, for the R who is answering the survey in Spanish, the first option is "Spanish only," whereas for the R who is answering in English the first option is "English only." In all versions, the "Spanish only" option is code 5 and the "English only" option is code 1.

● **Q49:** ***Highest grade of school completed.*** For this question, the interviewer must elicit the highest grade completed, which will present difficulties when R studied outside the U.S. educational system. Response categories must *not* be read aloud. If R offers as response the level of schooling completed, or degree or title obtained, the interviewer should probe for how many total years of schooling that level, degree, or title requires in the educational system in which R studied (i.e., how many years were required, starting with the first grade of primary school).

Spanish-language interviewers should be aware that the same label is used in different countries to refer to a different number of years of study. For example, *secundaria* denotes 9 years of schooling in Mexico, but 11 or 12 years in other countries. Likewise, *colegio* may refer to grade school in some countries, high school in others, and college in Puerto Rico.

▲ **Q50:** ***Annual household income.*** With this question, interviewers will find R's annual household income range by using a technique called *bracketing*. R is asked if income is less than $25,000, and, depending on the answer, follow-ups are used to ascertain higher or lower income until the proper range is coded. This response is recorded below the response categories, in a special two-digit box labeled "Code."

■ **Q51:** ***Sexual identification.*** This question is about self-identification, not sexual orientation or sexual activities. The interviewer should never paraphrase by asking, for example, whether R is attracted to, or has sex with, men or women. R may be married to someone of the opposite sex yet not self-identify as heterosexual.

In the cognitive testing, Spanish-speaking Rs were unsure whether *heterosexual, homosexual,* and *bisexual* corresponded with *straight, gay,* and *bisexual.* If R seems unsure of the meaning of the terms, or reluctant to select, the response is code 4. Code 7 applies only if R says he does not know, or is unsure of, which response option best describes him but seems to understand the terminology. The interviewer should not interpret or recode answers that are provided in terms completely different from the allowable response categories. For example, in cognitive testing, responses included, "I'm a man, a complete man." In such cases, the interviewer should reread the answer categories and ask R to select from the listed options.

● **Q52:** ***Current spouse or partner.*** Rs who supplied marital status earlier might find this question repetitive; the introduction acknowledges this repetition. This question is used to determine whether to ask the subsequent question.

● **Q53–54:** ***Spouse/partner's current and past tobacco use.*** Some Rs are not familiar with chewing or dipping tobacco.

● **Q55:** ***Zip code.*** Some Rs do not remember their zip code. This will not be a problem for in-person surveys: the interviewer will have R's address and the zip code can later be obtained. For telephone surveys, if no matching of phone numbers and addresses is planned, the interviewer may want to offer R a chance to ask someone else in the household for the zip code.

■ **Q56:** ***Health insurance coverage status.*** The qualifying sentence after the question is intended to exclude free or reduced-cost clinics for low-income Rs—clinics Latino Rs often use. The question pertains only to private or government-sponsored health coverage plans.

B.3 Optional Modules Q-by-Qs

The optional modules contain questions that can be used to supplement those in the core module. Although the core is the basic set of questions everyone should use for the H/L ATS, considerations of cost, time, and local interest will lead each surveying agency or organization to select some, all, or none of the questions in the optional modules.

Although Sections A to H are grouped into optional modules by topic, the questions in them do not have to be kept together, but instead may be inserted into sections of the core. Nor do they have to be placed in a core section named like the optional module. For instance, questions in the Detailed Demographics module ask about health; they could be integrated into Section 1 (General Health) in the core, while A1 might be best placed in Demographic Items (Section 6 of the core), near the education questions.

In adding questions from the optional modules to the core, the researcher must take care to modify skip instructions as appropriate. Each subset of questions in the optional modules is preceded by an indication of intended R type. In some instances, a subset of optional questions is preceded by a suggested placement in the core instrument.

Q-by-Qs are provided only for those questions that presented issues during cognitive testing.

Because the text of each question is not included in these Q-by-Qs, users of the guide may want to have a printout of the H/L ATS on hand:

- H/L ATS Optional Modules (in English)
- H/L ATS Optional Modules (Spanish, with English Instructions for Programmers and Interviewers)
- H/L ATS Preguntas adicionales (totalmente en español)

B.3.1 Section A: Detailed Demographic Items

The supplemental Demographic Items section consists of three questions (QA1 to QA3): one on current enrollment in an educational program (QA1) and two on health problems or impairments (QA2 and QA3).

▲ **QA3:** ***Health problems requiring use of special equipment.*** As indicated in the questionnaire, if R reports using special equipment on occasion, the code is "Yes."

B.3.2 Section B: Detailed Tobacco Use Questions

The supplemental Tobacco Use section consists of 15 questions (QB1 to QB15) that focus on smoking initiation in young adults, smoking patterns, brand use, purchase patterns, use of other tobacco products (such as smokeless tobacco products, cigars, pipes, bidis, kreteks, and new tobacco products), and intention to smoke for young adults who are not current smokers.

■ **QB8a:** ***Buying cigarettes in a neighboring state.*** In cognitive testing it was observed that many Rs, particularly but not exclusively recent immigrants, had a limited geographic sense. Some named other cities or counties as neighboring states. The interviewer therefore should identify neighboring states for R. Neighboring states include only U.S. states, not Mexican states or Canadian provinces.

▲ **QB9a–b:** ***Smokeless tobacco products.*** Rs may not know what snuff is. None of the Rs in the cognitive tests had heard of snuff. No definition is provided. Even Rs who do not know what snuff is will understand the term *smokeless tobacco products;* use of this term will not compromise their responses.

▲ **QB10a:** ***Cigars.*** There are multiple terms used in Latin America to refer to cigars. In cognitive testing it was determined that, despite the multiplicity of terms, all Rs understood the term *puro* as cigar.

▲ **QB12a–13b:** ***Kreteks or bidis.*** Rs may not know what kreteks and bidis are. None of the Rs in the cognitive tests had heard of them. A definition of the word *bidis* appears in the question stem, and an alternative name appears for *kreteks* in the question itself. Code 7 if the R states he does not know what kreteks or bidis are.

B.3.3 Section C: Detailed Cessation Questions

The supplemental Cessation section consists of 10 questions (QC1 to QC10) that focus on smoking cessation, including interest in quitting, dentist's advice for quitting, medications R used to quit, and methods other than medication that R used to quit.

There are no Q-by-Qs for this module. The intent of the questions and the vocabulary were clear to our test participants.

B.3.4 Section D: Detailed Environmental Tobacco Smoke Questions

This Environmental Tobacco Smoke section consists of 10 questions (QD1 to QD10) about workplace smoking, attitudes regarding policies for clean indoor air, and behavior regarding clean indoor air.

▲ **QD2:** ***Attitude about smoking in bars.*** For the Spanish versions, optional terms for bars and cocktail lounges are offered to cover terminology used in different countries. In cognitive testing it was determined that "bares, barras, cantinas, o taberna" was a phrase generally understood by all. It clearly identified drinking establishments, although the clientele for each of these places varies by country.

■ **QD6–7:** ***Avoidance of restaurants because smoking is or is not permitted.*** Because these two items sound alike, the R might think the interviewer is repeating the same question. The interviewer should stress the word *not* in D7 to avoid this error.

B.3.5 Section E: Health and Social Influences

This Health and Social Influences section contains 10 questions (QE1 to QE10) about the health effects of smoking, smoking-related conditions that the R may have been diagnosed with, additional risk perceptions, and peer and family influences for and against smoking.

There are no Q-by-Qs for this module. The intent of the questions and the vocabulary were clear to our test participants.

B.3.6 Section F: Policy Issues

The Policy Issues section consists of eight questions (QF1 to QF8) covering opinions on youth tobacco use, sponsoring and marketing of tobacco products, and taxation of cigarette sales.

▲ **QF1:** ***Community prevention of sales of tobacco to teens.*** This item is intended to elicit R's views on his local community's role in preventing sales of tobacco to minors.

● **QF6:** ***Monetary donations from tobacco companies.*** In this question both donations and contributions should be understood as *monetary* and not as donations of tobacco products.

■ **QF8:** ***Support for levels of taxation on cigarettes.*** This is a dense question that Rs in cognitive testing found difficult to process. Interviewers should read the item slowly, giving Rs the opportunity to process the information.

B.3.7 Section G: Parental Involvement

The nine questions in the Parental Involvement section (QG1 to QG9) apply only to parents of children aged 5 to 17 years. They cover parent-child communication about tobacco use, Rs' parental beliefs about their children's smoking status, disapproval Rs would feel if their children smoked, and curfew for Rs' children.

▲ **QG1:** ***Age of child nearest age 10 in R's household.*** This question is used to determine on which child the subsequent questions in Section G will focus. As indicated before the question, if two children are equally close to age 10, the older child should be selected. In the case of twins, the firstborn child should be selected.

B.3.8 Section H: Media Exposure

This section consists of three questions about how much exposure the R has had to commercials or messages promoting smoking or not smoking in the 7 days preceding the interview.

There are no Q-by-Qs for this module. The intent of the questions and the vocabulary were clear to our test participants.

B.4 Screeners

The H/L ATS Screener is a brief script with a sequence of questions to be asked of the household respondent. Its purpose is to determine (1) the eligibility of a household to participate in the H/L ATS and (2) which household member should be interviewed. There are two versions: one for a telephone survey and one for a face-to-face survey:

- Telephone Screener (English)
- In-person Screener (English)
- Telephone Screener (Spanish, with English Instructions for Programmers and Interviewers)
- In-person Screener (Spanish, with English Instructions for Programmers and Interviewers)
- "Cuestionario de selección" por teléfono (totalmente en español)
- "Cuestionario de selección" cara-a-cara (totalmente en español)

The telephone and in-person screeners are very similar to one another, and they are both patterned on the screener used for the General Population State ATS.

The telephone screener is used to accomplish the following:

- Verify that the telephone number belongs to a household (not to a business or institution).
- Ask if anyone in the household is Hispanic or Latino.
- Obtain a count of all Hispanic or Latino adult household members by gender.
- Perform a random selection from among these eligible Rs.

The result of the random selection by telephone screener is communicated to the household respondent as a combination of birth order and gender. For example, the interviewer may say he needs to speak with "the oldest male" or "the fifth-oldest female" (the designation is made by the computer). Once the selected individual is reached, the screener is used to verify the person's Hispanic or Latino ethnicity, elicit national origin, and ask if he prefers to be interviewed in English or in Spanish.

The face-to-face screener is used to accomplish the following:

- Verify that the interviewer is at the sampled address.
- Ask if anyone in the household is Hispanic or Latino.

- Obtain a count of all Hispanic or Latino adult household members by gender.
- Perform a random selection from among these eligible Rs.

The result of the random selection by face-to-face screener is communicated to the household respondent as a combination of birth order and gender. For example, the interviewer may say he needs to speak with "the oldest male" or "the fifth-oldest female," depending on what the random table indicates. For face-to-face interviews conducted by paper and pencil, the interviewer will follow a protocol provided by the research director to randomly select one of the combinations. Once the selected individual is reached, the screener is used to verify the person's Hispanic or Latino ethnicity, elicit national origin, and ask whether he prefers to be interviewed in English or in Spanish.

B.5 Advance Letters

Advance letters are mailed to addresses of households selected to participate in a survey. The purpose of these letters is to introduce the survey to the sampled households and alert them that they will be contacted. In surveys of Hispanic populations, advance letters are a particularly important means of providing legitimacy to the study and improving cooperation (Carley-Baxter, Link, Roe, & Quiroz, 2006).

In Latino households, an unannounced visit or telephone call tends to generate suspicion, especially in households with limited English language or in households that include undocumented immigrants. As an interview medium, the telephone is viewed negatively, described as cold, and "generally seen with suspicion, possibly because of fraud and scams done by telemarketers" (Schoua-Glusberg, 2000). Telephone survey response rates among Latinos have been shown to be significantly higher when an advance letter is used than when it is not (Carley-Baxter et al., 2006).

The following letters were prepared as part of the H/L ATS survey materials (Appendices A–D).

- Advance Letter to Potential Households, Telephone Survey (English)
- Advance Letter to Potential Households, Telephone Survey (Spanish)
- Advance Letter to Potential Households, In-person Survey (English)
- Advance Letter to Potential Households, In-person Survey (Spanish)

An advance letter usually includes an explanation of the survey, identification of the sponsoring organization, the purpose of collecting the data, and an explanation of how the data will be used. It also includes a message about the voluntary nature of survey participation, the ability of the R to skip questions he does not want to answer, and an assurance of the security of the data. Finally, if the survey offers any compensation for R's time, monetary or otherwise, it is mentioned in the letter. Recipients are provided with a means of contacting the sponsoring or data-collection organization. Advance letters generally aid in increasing survey participation and in reducing the number of contacts required to obtain a full response to the survey (Dillman, 2000).

Generally an advance letter is mailed within 2 weeks of making first contact with a sampled household. If mailed too early, it likely will have been forgotten by the time the household is contacted for the interview. Mailed too close to the contact date, it may not yet have been received or read.

If the survey uses a random-digit-dial sample, the survey organization should attempt to match each telephone number selected with its corresponding mailing address in order to send the advance letter. This objective can be achieved with use of one of multiple commercial services that provide this kind of matching. Not all phone numbers will be successfully matched, however: interviewers should be aware that a household they contact might never have received the advance letter.

Even when address matching is successful, it is possible that no name of householders is available. In this case, the letter will often be addressed to the household without naming any specific person. Because this method is not as effective as an individually addressed letter, it is important to ensure that the outside of the envelope looks like an important communication, one not easily confused with "junk mail."

Because some Rs will not have received the letter, will have forgotten it, or will have had someone else in the household read it instead, the telephone interviewer will have to be prepared for Rs who ask to see something in writing before they agree to participate. Procedures must be in place to mail new copies of the advance letter to households requesting it.

For face-to-face surveys, interviewers will carry with them a copy of the advance letter to provide to participants who request one. Alternatively, if the sample for a face-to-face survey is geographically clustered, interviewers may distribute advance letters under doors in selected addresses in their area before they start ringing any doorbells. This approach has proved successful in other area probability surveys involving a large percentage of Latino households (Schoua-Glusberg, 1998).

If the survey uses a list sample—that is, one by which individuals are selected instead of addresses or phone numbers—the letters and envelopes should be personalized.

B.6 Informed Consent Text and Forms

Informed consent forms serve two important purposes.[1] First, they are designed to fully inform prospective survey Rs about what they are being asked to do, why the research is necessary and important, what participation actually entails, how their privacy and security will be protected, and the risks or benefits attending their participation. Rs are provided with

[1] The consent form and consent text provided here differ slightly from those used in the Centers for Disease Control and Prevention's 2007 survey.

a means of contacting someone who can answer questions about their rights as participants in a survey. The goal is to ensure that participants' rights are protected and that when they agree to participate they do so with a clear understanding of what will be involved.

The second purpose of an informed consent form is to protect the survey organization and survey sponsor from any future claims that the participant was unaware of either what participation would entail or the benefits or risks he would or could experience.

In face-to-face surveys, the consent form is read by (or to) the R, who must sign it before the interview can begin. If the R agrees to the consent form but does not want to sign his name (perhaps for reasons of confidentiality), the protocol approved by the study's institutional review board for such situations should be followed (Appendices E and F):

- Informed Consent Form, In-person Survey (English)
- Informed Consent Form, In-person Survey (Spanish)

In telephone surveys a consent text is read by the telephone interviewer; the participant gives verbal agreement instead of a signature (Appendices G and H):

- Informed Consent Text, Telephone Survey (English)
- Informed Consent Text, Telephone Survey (Spanish)

In either case, if the R does not agree, the interviewer must politely terminate the interview and not ask any additional questions.

Low-literacy populations may have problems reading and interpreting the written consent form. To make the situation less awkward, the interviewer may say, "I'm going to read this to you, unless you prefer to read it yourself." It is important that interviewers be able to explain terms in the letter and respond to any questions the R might have. Interviewers should pay attention to verbal and nonverbal indications that the R may be having difficulty understanding what he is reading or hearing.

C. SAMPLING AND WEIGHTING

In this section we examine issues that were considered in developing the sample designs for the three Hispanic/Latino Adult Tobacco Survey (H/L ATS) case study sites. The important lesson is not how these issues were resolved in the three case studies, but how these issues relate to the population of interest. Most of these issues will be relevant in sampling other Hispanic and Latino target populations. It is recommended that a sampling statistician be consulted when the sampling plan for a specific survey is designed.

C.1 Sampling in Three Case Study Surveys

Three case studies are presented here that illustrate different approaches to developing probability samples of the Hispanic and Latino population. The three areas chosen for the case studies are (1) four boroughs of New York City; (2) Miami-Dade County, Florida; and (3) a compact group of three Hispanic neighborhoods called *colonias* in El Paso County, Texas, along the Texas-Mexico border. These locations were selected in part because they are typical of many such communities across the country; therefore, survey and sampling approaches that work in these three locations should work similarly in corresponding areas.

The main differences between the three surveys involve the mode of data collection and the recommended sampling frame. For determining the best mode of data collection for each area (telephone versus in-person), a crucial consideration is the percentage of the target area that is Hispanic. The New York case study represents a highly urban area with a slightly above-average density of Hispanic or Latino persons (29%). Miami, Florida, is likewise an urban area, but the density is notably higher (57%).

Both New York and Miami-Dade case studies target larger geographic areas with a smaller percentage of Hispanic persons than the *colonias*; therefore, a substantial number of households must be screened in these areas to locate Hispanic respondents. Telephone interviewing of a sample chosen from a standard list-assisted random-digit-dial (RDD) frame of telephone numbers is the choice for New York and Miami (Casady & Lepkowski, 1991) because in these sites (1) most households have telephone service and (2) the Hispanic and Latino population is relatively spread out. Telephone interviewing means there will be no interviewer travel costs and screening can be done efficiently.

By contrast, of the three case study areas, the *colonias* have the highest density of Hispanic and Latino persons (96%). Area sampling and face-to-face interviewing of selected residential dwellings is the choice for the *colonias* (Kish, 1965): many households there lack home telephones; the population resides in a small, contained area; and many persons there speak only Spanish. Face-to-face screening (area sampling) and in-person interviewing, therefore, should yield a better response rate than telephone interviewing. Moreover, this approach is relatively cost-efficient because sampling a compact area means interviewer travel cost will be low.

All survey research plans in all three sites share the following features:

- The sampling approach proposed for each site provides for a probability sample that can be considered representative of the target population.
- The sample frame of households developed in each site is random and representative.
- The target population for each survey is Hispanic/Latino residents aged 18 years or older and located by screening the households in the sample.
- The research objective of each survey is to profile patterns of adult tobacco use in the target population.
- The same survey materials are used in each site (with minor differences to accommodate the different modes of data collection).
- Targeted sample size in each location is 1,500 respondents, with one adult randomly selected from each sampled household.
- Respondents must speak either English or Spanish.

Table C-1. Description of the Three H/L ATS Case Study Sites

Case study site	Approximate Hispanic adult pop. (year 2000)	Approximate Hispanic adult pop. (%)	Sampling frame(s)	Mode of data collection
New York City: boroughs of Brooklyn, Bronx, Manhattan, and Queens	1,227,200	29	List-assisted RDD	Telephone
Florida: the Miami portion of Dade County	971,800	57	List-assisted RDD	Telephone
El Paso County, Texas: *colonias* named Clint, San Elizario, and Socorro	23,500	96	List of U.S. Census blocks: lists residential dwellings in each sample block	In-person

C.1.1 New York, New York: Telephone Survey in Urban Area with Moderate Concentration of Hispanic and Latino Persons

New York's is a stratified simple random sample of enough telephone numbers to yield about 1,500 completed interviews with self-identified Hispanic residents aged 18 or older who can be reached by landline telephone in the four targeted boroughs of the Bronx, Brooklyn, Manhattan, and Queens.[2] For a site like New York, with its large area and low

[2] Limiting sampling to those households with telephone access creates some coverage bias in that it excludes Hispanic households without a home phone (Lessler & Kalsbeek, 1992). This source of bias can usually be controlled somewhat through weights calibration, by *poststratifying,* or *raking,* the weights as mentioned in Section C.3.3 (Kalton & Flores-Cervantes, 2003).

concentration of Hispanic and Latino persons, the topics that follow address increase of efficiency in the sampling approach and minimization of the costs of screening for Hispanic and Latino households.

Geographic Constraints

The New York case study targets the four New York boroughs with the highest density of Hispanic and Latino households. In this case, the researchers were satisfied that representative findings based on these four boroughs would meet their needs.

Use of List-assisted RDD

A list-assisted RDD telephone sample frame was recommended for New York. A list-assisted frame typically consists of those telephone numbers in telephone 100-banks[3] with at least one directory-listed telephone number (*list-assisted* because directory listings help identify the telephone prefixes to be sampled). List-assisted RDD sampling is recommended over other methods for several important reasons. List-assisted RDD sampling is more efficient than straight RDD sampling (choosing 10-digit phone numbers completely at random within the target area) because the list will contain a higher percentage of residential telephone numbers, and therefore less effort will be spent dialing nonproductive numbers. Sampling directly from a telephone directory would certainly result in more residential numbers, but it would exclude unlisted and unpublished phone numbers, a potentially serious source of bias (Kalsbeek & Agans, 2007). Similarly, Spanish surname lists drawn from published directories or other sources typically have limited coverage, which reduces the representativeness of the population. None of the three case studies recommends the use of surname lists.

Oversampling

Even after sampling is limited to these four boroughs, only 29% of the households contacted are expected to be Hispanic or Latino. A significant portion of the calling effort will have to be devoted to household screening. To improve these odds, it is possible to *oversample* Hispanic populations by identifying telephone prefixes known to contain higher concentrations of Hispanic households and sampling from these prefixes at a higher rate (Kalsbeek & Agans, 2007).

At the borough level, the percentage of Hispanic persons in the population for the Bronx (57%) is roughly twice that in the other boroughs (20%, 27%, and 26% for Brooklyn, Manhattan, and Queens, respectively). Oversampling phone numbers from the Bronx, therefore, may improve the calling efficiency for Hispanic households. To further increase the calling efficiency, oversampling by borough can be combined with oversampling of telephone prefixes known to correspond with higher concentrations of Hispanic households. These increases in calling efficiency come at a price, though, in terms of loss of precision

[3] A *100-bank* consists of those telephone numbers with the same first 8 digits of a 10-digit number.

(because of variable sampling probabilities and weights; Kalsbeek, 2003). The optimal allocation of sample between these methods also depends on the goals of the survey (e.g., whether separate estimates are sought for individual boroughs). Determining optimal sampling rates requires careful consideration of both statistical and practical implications. It is recommended that a sampling statistician and survey methodologist confer to discuss the pros and cons of any specific situation (Cochran, 1977).

Determining the Number of Selected Phone Numbers to Call

Although the telephone survey designs for New York and Florida target 1,500 completed interviews, the actual number of sample phone numbers that have to be called is much greater. The experience of prior telephone surveys with similar topics, target populations, or sample recruitment strategies can help with estimating the quantity of phone numbers that will be required. If Y is the expected ratio of number of respondents to number of assigned phone numbers, accounting for all sources of attrition combined, then to obtain 1,500 respondents one must assign $1{,}500/Y$ for calling in the site. When attrition patterns are likely to differ among the sampling strata that are used, one should separately estimate sample attrition and the number of selected phone numbers in each stratum or groups of strata where attrition is expected to be similar.

C.1.2 Miami, Florida: Telephone Survey in Urban Area with Higher Concentration of Hispanic and Latino Persons

Oversampling will result in some loss of precision; therefore, the value of oversampling areas with relatively high Hispanic concentrations must be balanced against the loss of precision due to variable weights (Kalsbeek, 2003). Because Miami has a greater concentration of Hispanic persons to begin with (57% as opposed to New York's 29%), a simpler sampling plan—just oversampling telephone prefixes with higher concentrations of Hispanic households—is recommended.

In both of these examples, the sole purpose of sample stratification is to facilitate an oversampling of Hispanic persons in the target area. Investigators may also be concerned about the precision of the estimate of tobacco use. If there is a large difference in the tobacco use levels between different parts of the target population, it may be of value to incorporate this information into the sampling plan. The merits of different sampling rates in a multistrata design would have to be evaluated by a sampling statistician in light of the specific characteristics of the target population. Suggested approaches for determining optimal sample allocations in different situations are provided in Section F.2: References and Resources.

C.1.3 El Paso, Texas: In-person Survey in Border Areas with High Concentration of Hispanic and Latino Persons

Multistage area sampling is commonly used to select households in face-to-face sample surveys, such as that for the El Paso site (see Kish, 1965). Area samples are most useful when the target area of the survey can be subdivided into a reasonably large number of well-defined geopolitical subunits for which population counts, maps, and other statistical data are available.

Two plausible alternatives to area sampling rely on different frame sources. One is sampling directly from postal mailing lists of residences (Iannacchione, Staab, & Redden, 2003), and the other is sampling parcels of land via electronic property tax files (Kalsbeek, Kavanagh, & Wu, 2004). Both of these alternatives have been shown to generate samples with very good coverage, to be simple and inexpensive to use, and to avoid the usually negative statistical effects of cluster sampling. Mailing lists have the added advantage of an easily accessible mailing address for sending advance letters, and the tax parcel approach has the added benefit of latitude-longitude coordinates to make sampled parcels easier to find.

Deciding on Sampling Units

Selection of an area sample of Hispanic persons in a local setting like the *colonias* typically calls for first choosing a sample of area subunits as primary sampling units (PSUs) and then randomly selecting a sample of residential dwellings as secondary sampling units (SSUs) in each selected PSU.[4] Each sample PSU is best chosen with a probability proportional to its size (i.e., a PPS, with *size* referring to the best measure of the number of Hispanic households in the PSU). An approximately equal number of Hispanic dwellings are then chosen within each PSU. The chosen dwellings come from a list frame separately and specially constructed by trained field staff who follow a rigorous protocol for list construction. The Census block is the most practical PSU for the H/L ATS in the El Paso site because (1) there are a sufficient number of them, (2) they are a tier of aggregation for urban sociodemographic characteristics from the decennial Census, and (3) there exist block maps with well-defined boundaries to facilitate sampling of dwellings within blocks.

Deciding on the Allocation Among Sampling Stages

A key feature of a multistage household sample is the allocation of the sample among stages. This allocation for the two-stage household sample design in the El Paso site is determined by the number of sample blocks (PSUs) and the average number of *selected* dwellings per sample PSU. These numbers are determined so that the total number of *responding* households will be 1,500. The experience of previously completed surveys can

[4] The terms *dwelling, housing unit, dwelling unit,* and *household* are synonymous, with the first three terms referring to the place where a group of related or unrelated individuals (comprising the household) resides.

help guide the decision about the number of selected dwellings to use as compared with the number of responding households required.

A good rule to follow is, the greater the number of sample PSUs one can afford, the better the statistical results from the sample will be. In practical terms, most good samples of this type strive for at least 50 sample PSUs and an average number of responding households per PSU no greater than 30.

Identifying Sampling Strata

Because the concentration of Hispanic persons is uniformly high in all three *colonias*, oversampling them by disproportionately sampling among *colonias* would not make household screening notably more efficient. However, PSU stratification by *colonia* would improve the precision of estimates of smoking prevalence for the population of Hispanic adults in the three *colonias* combined if there were substantial differences in smoking behavior among *colonias*.[5] The greater these differences, the greater the statistical benefit.

Stratification by other block-level characteristics available from the 2000 Census may also slightly improve the precision of H/L ATS estimates if those characteristics are correlated with smoking behavior measures of interest. Gender and other known predictors of smoking behavior that are available from Census block-level summary data could be used for this purpose.

Allocating Sample Size for Blocks Among Strata

Allocation of the sample of blocks among the PSU sampling strata will depend on which domains of the population are most important for analysis findings. If *colonias* and one or more other block-level characteristics are used to define strata, if the most important survey estimates are smoking prevalence rates for all Hispanic adults in the three *colonias* combined, and if the rates are not dramatically different among strata, then a proportionate allocation of the sample of blocks is the best choice. If, on the other hand, comparison of estimates among *colonias* is the highest priority, one third of the sample of blocks should be allocated to each of the *colonias,* and then the equal *colonia* sample sizes should be proportionately allocated among the strata within each *colonia*.

Selecting PPS Sample of Census Blocks as PSUs

An equal-probability sample of households, and its associated benefits, can be achieved within each stratum of a two-stage design (Kish, 1965). This outcome is accomplished by selection of blocks (PSUs) with PPS, with the best estimate of current household size as the size measure for PPS selection, and then selection of an equal number of dwellings within each selected block. A number of PPS selection methods could be used in this circumstance. One approach is PPS systematic sampling in which the PPS selection rule is applied to a

---

[5] Data from the 2000 Census indicates that for the *colonias* the percentage of the population that is Hispanic is 97.9% in San Elizario, 84.0% in Clint, and 96.4% in Socorro.

strategically ordered PSU frame by using a systematically selected sequence of numbers. Two alternatives are PPS with replacement sampling, in which it is possible to select a PSU multiple times, and PPS without replacement sampling, in which repeat selection is not allowed (Cochran, 1977). Each approach has its merits; these merits would have to be evaluated by a sampling statistician familiar with the specific target population.

Constructing a Sampling Frame for Second-stage Sampling

Choosing a subsample of dwellings may not be necessary in some sample blocks. When the average number of dwellings per block is small (e.g., fewer than 20), it may be more practical to include all dwellings in the SSU sample. The cutoff for identifying sample blocks not requiring subsampling depends on the targeted average number of responding households per sample PSU.

In those sample blocks where a subsample of dwellings is chosen, the frame for choosing dwellings may be constructed in a number of ways. The traditional approach has been to train field staff to list all dwellings by following a predetermined path around the boundary and internal streets of the block group. Although this approach produces a useful frame, it is relatively expensive to implement. Publicly available postal mailing lists and property tax parcel listings are alternatives.

Selecting Sample of Dwellings Within PSUs

Simple random sampling is typically applied to the block-specific frames just described. As with telephone sampling, the number of selected households in this final stage of household sampling must account for sample attrition due to ineligibility (e.g., vacant dwelling) and other reasons for nonresponse (e.g., refusal, not at home, unavailable) to result in 1,500 participating households.

C.2 Within-household Sampling

Households in H/L ATS samples are clusters of one or more Hispanic adults. One resident is randomly chosen for the survey interview in each household. Although there are several alternative methods for randomly choosing the resident, the H/L ATS screener employs the "*n*th-oldest adult" approach. This approach is relatively easy to use and is generally noninvasive, especially as compared with the household roster approach, though it can somewhat skew the sample.[6]

In its simplest version, the *n*th-oldest adult approach begins by determining the number of Hispanic adults residing in the household and then chooses a random number between one

[6] Some surveys request specific identifying information (e.g., the selected resident's first name or gender and age) to form a detailed household roster to use as the basis for resident selection. This is preferred from a technical standpoint to reduce gender bias, but asking for more clearly identifying information on a household roster in this way increasingly has been seen by respondents as prying or intrusive and has led to higher refusal rates. The H/L ATS screener does not use this method.

and the number of reported residents. The selected resident is designated by age, relative to the oldest resident. For example, if there are three eligible adults and the number 2 is randomly chosen, then the second-oldest adult is interviewed.

C.2.1 Reducing Gender Bias in Respondent Selection

The *n*th-oldest, next/last-birthday, and other respondent-selection methods that choose a resident at random often lead to a gender bias favoring females in the composition of the final respondent sample, if the gender of the selected resident is not provided. For example, populations with 50:50 splits between males and females can lead to 40:60 or even 30:70 splits in the respondent sample. One reason for this gender imbalance is that, all else being constant, females are more likely than males to be available for and respond to interview surveys. Another explanation for this gender imbalance is the tendency for the household resident completing the screener (more likely female than male) to claim to be the selected respondent if the selection method does not explicitly indicate who is to be chosen (Carr & Hertvik, 1993; Oldendick, Bishop, Sorenson, & Tuchfarber, 1988).

Gender bias can be reduced by more explicitly specifying who is selected. The H/L ATS screener asks for the number of adult Hispanic males and adult Hispanic females in the household. The interviewer can, for example, ask for the oldest female. With this approach, it is typical to require a separate random (i.e., Poisson) sampling decision for each household member, using selection probabilities that vary by subgroup characteristic (Lohr, 1999).

C.2.2 Respondent Selection in Multifamily Hispanic Households

In border areas like the *colonias,* there may be a higher frequency of multifamily households in the heavily Hispanic neighborhoods. Recently immigrated families tend to move in with more established residents, live with relatives, or "double up" with other recently immigrated families. A decision should be made early about whether the survey will recognize multiple families as separate sampling units or treat the sum of all adult residents as a single family for sampling purposes.

If the sum of adults is treated as a single family, the screener respondent must "count up" the total number of adults in residence, and then a single person is selected. Alternatively, multiple families at a single address may be considered separate reporting units for study data collection and therefore may be treated in effect as separate households. There are two options in this case: one is to conduct an interview with each family; the other is to first randomly choose one of the families and then select a respondent from among the residents of the selected family.

Selecting only one family avoids any estimate precision loss otherwise due to the clustering effect of interviewing multiple residents from the same household, but it can also contribute to reduced precision due to increased variation in selection probabilities among respondents. Furthermore, selecting one family and one respondent avoids the practical difficulty of coding response dispositions from two respondents in the same household. Finally, allowing for multiple respondents per household makes it harder to predict how many interviews the sample will yield.

C.2.3 Additional Considerations

Two remaining points should be kept in mind. First, within-household sampling is another stage in the sample design. The probability of inclusion for any sample member in multistage designs is the product of selection probabilities for sample outcomes in each stage leading to the choosing of that member. The approach followed in selecting persons to interview is critical to determining the selection probabilities required to produce sample weights.

Second, in a computer-assisted telephone survey, the system will automatically choose whom to ask for, in accordance with the answers to screening questions. Operationalizing sampling procedures in an in-person screening, though, can be difficult. Interviewers must be provided a clear, easy-to-follow protocol for deciding what *n* is when they ask for the *n*th-oldest adult, man or woman.

C.3 Weighting Methods in the Three H/L ATS Case studies

During analysis, formulas are applied to sample data to produce estimates of the population characteristics. The statistical quality (or accuracy) of any survey estimate is measured by the size of its mean-squared error, which jointly depends on the precision (measured by variance or standard error of the estimate) and the bias of the estimate. Statistical inference based on probability samples offers an added advantage over inference using nonprobability samples: the analyst, using data from the chosen sample, can directly obtain measures of the statistical precision of estimates, although, like the survey estimates, these measures of precision are also estimates. These precision measures are required in order to produce confidence intervals, tests of hypothesis, and other statistical products of analysis. To supplement efforts called for by the survey design, the bias of survey estimates must be measured.

Appropriately estimating population characteristics and their precision requires that design features such as stratification, cluster sampling, and numerical measures of variable selection probabilities (i.e., leading to the computation of sample weights) be accommodated in analysis. Lohr (1999) offers a relatively recent review of the general design strategies and estimation issues related to sampling from finite populations. A more thorough discussion of other design issues in telephone surveys is given by Kalsbeek and Agans (2007). The representativeness of the selected sample may be altered by limitations in the selection and data-gathering processes, including frames that selectively cover the target population, and differential nonresponse by members of the selected sample and among data items sought from responding sample members (Lessler & Kalsbeek, 1992).

C.3.1 Sample Weights

To produce representative findings, the analyst should (1) compute sampling weights to account for the process of sample selection and important composition-altering forces at work on the sample during the sampling and data collection processes, and (2) in analysis use statistical formulations that utilize these weights and appropriately account for stratification and cluster sampling in generating survey findings.

A sample weight is a statistical measurement linked to a data record for any survey respondent. In general terms, it is computed as the inverse of the adjusted probability of obtaining the data for the respondent. In most cases this probability is simply the respondent's original selection probability based on the sample design. The inverse probability, or base weight, is often adjusted to account for unintended sample imbalance arising during the conduction of the survey. More than one weight adjustment may be applied, and all are multiplicative.

Unless a weight is rescaled for analytic purposes (e.g., normalized to sum to the number of sample respondents), its value can be interpreted as an indication of the number of population members represented by the respondent. Separate sets of weights may be necessary when data are gathered for different types of data items associated with the respondent. For example, if data in a household survey are gathered for the selected households and for one resident chosen at random in each of those households, a separate set of weights is produced for the household data and the resident data.

C.3.2 Weight Calculation

Some combination of the following steps is typically followed to produce from a probability sample a set of weights for the "*i*th" individual-respondent data record, with the final adjusted weight being the product of the value generated in each step. If at all possible, all of the following steps should be completed on H/L ATS survey samples:

1. Base weight (determined by the probability of choosing the household and the method of respondent selection within the household).
2. Adjustment for nonresponse (to partially offset the biasing effects of differential response rates in the sample).
3. Adjustment for incomplete sample coverage (to partially correct for any bias due to differential coverage of the population by the list or lists from which the sample is chosen).
4. Adjustment to control variation among weights (to limit the loss in the precision of survey estimates due to widely variable sample weights).
5. Adjustment to calibrate the weights to the sampled population (to compensate for any sample imbalance not accommodated by the other adjustments).

Step 1 must always be completed in H/L ATS samples described in the case studies. For it to be completed, the sample design must qualify as a probability sample design, and steps followed in selecting the sample must be well documented so that selection probabilities can be determined for each survey respondent. Step 2 may be done if the sample can be subdivided into subgroups among which survey response rates differ. Step 3 will almost never be used for H/L ATS samples: computing it is practical only for sites where telephone sampling is done *and* for which there are external data on households with and without telephone access. Step 4 is particularly important in sites where the sample is significantly disproportionate (e.g., as a result of efforts to oversample Hispanic households). Step 5 is both important and difficult to implement for the typical target population of the H/L ATS.

C.3.3 Lack of Known Totals to Calibrate Weights

Step 5, sometimes referred to as *weighting up to known totals,* is a final correction that helps make the weighted data more representative of the target population. Weights calibration, however, requires high-quality external data on the target population distribution by population characteristics highly correlated with adult smoking behavior. Large, national-level population surveys commonly rely on information obtained from the most recent decennial Census, the Current Population Survey, or the American Community Survey. As the three case studies suggest, the H/L ATS is typically conducted at the substate, and often subcounty, level. It can be difficult to find a data source sufficiently current and of high quality to use in calibrating weights for a specific target population. Data from the most recent decennial Census are usually the best available option, although Census counts may not be altogether current.

Even if such data are available for a specific area, they may lack sufficient detail to correctly weight the data, as explained in the *Assessment of Major Federal Data Sets for Analyses of Hispanic and Asian or Pacific Islander Subgroups and Native Americans:*

> All of the major surveys use poststratification in the final stage of weighting to reduce sampling errors, and to compensate as much as possible for nonresponse and undercoverage. There are almost always separate poststratification cells for blacks, Hispanics, and all other race/ethnic groups. . . . The minority subgroups are almost always combined into categories like "total Hispanics" or "total other races. . . ." Subdomains such as Puerto-Ricans, Cuban-Americans, Central-Americans, etc., are thus combined into a single class, with identical weights. . . . If, in fact, some of these subgroups have lower response rates than the overall rate for the race/ethnic class, and are not separately adjusted, they will be underrepresented in the statistics. A similar situation exists with undercoverage. For example, if illegal aliens tend to avoid reporting (as seems likely) and if a higher proportion of Mexican-Americans are here illegally than in other Hispanic subpopulations (as is also likely), then the uniform weighting will slightly understate Mexican-Americans and overstate other Hispanic subgroups. (Waksberg, Levine, & Marker, 2000, sec. 2.7)

This statement is both an argument for achieving the highest response rates possible and a caveat about using known totals to weight the data.

C.3.4 Statistical Software for Complex Survey Designs

The sampling approaches described in the case studies are considered complex in that they may involve cluster selection, stratification, and sample weights. To prepare weights and weighted estimates from complex designs, one does best to use statistical software packages that rely on approximation or replication-based methods to estimate the variance of estimates (Wolter, 1985). A listing and several reviews of computer software that accommodates the sample design in this way are available online from the Survey Research Methods Section of the American Statistical Association at http://www.hcp.med.harvard.edu/statistics/survey-soft/.

D. ANALYSIS AND REPORTING

Surveillance of tobacco use and related attitudes, knowledge, and beliefs is key to promoting reductions in tobacco use in Hispanic and Latino communities. Research has shown that well-conducted tobacco surveys that preserve the privacy of respondents produce reliable and accurate findings. Over the years, epidemiologists have developed effective questions, scales, and indices for measuring tobacco behaviors, attitudes, and beliefs. With good sample design, survey methodology, and survey execution, results from the Hispanic/Latino Adult Tobacco Survey (H/L ATS) can improve the ability to track tobacco use, knowledge, attitudes, and beliefs in a specific study population.

Four examples of analysis and reporting are provided in this guide (Sections D.1 through D.4). The behavior and policy outcomes used in these examples were chosen because they directly speak to the Centers for Disease Control and Prevention's and the Office on Smoking and Health's goals to (1) reduce initiation, (2) reduce exposure to secondhand smoke among nonsmokers, and (3) increase cessation.

For each of these three major goals, one can track survey data over time to assess the population of interest. Such assessment may consist of comparing this population with other populations, identifying necessary intervention programs, developing health messages and other social marketing communications, and tracking the effectiveness of programs.

Each of the Sections D.1 through D.4 begins by identifying the variables used to address the topic at hand. Variables are divided between "outcome" measures (the behavior to be explained) and "domain" measures (the factors used to predict the behavior). The variables are identified by question number from the H/L ATS.

The variables analyzed in Sections D.1 through D.4 illustrate how these four topics might be addressed. They are not intended to be an exhaustive treatment of analysis and reporting possibilities for the H/L ATS.

D.1 Tobacco Use Among Young Adults

Tobacco use among young adults is a critical item of information for crafting tobacco cessation and tobacco use avoidance programs. Section D.1 identifies some H/L ATS items that may be used to describe tobacco use among young adults in the target population. Table D-1 summarizes the questionnaire items that are used in the analysis tables (Tables D-2 through D-7).

Table D-1. H/L ATS Questions Addressed in Tables D-2 Through D-7

Variable	Table D-2	Table D-3	Table D-4	Table D-5	Table D-6	Table D-7
Outcomes	Q2, Q4, Q5	Q2, Q4, Q5, Q6, Q7	Q2, Q4	Q2, Q4, Q5	Q2, Q3	Q10
Domains	Q41, Q45	Q41, Q45	Q41	Q41, Q45, Q46	Q41, Q49, Q49a	Q2, Q4, Q5, Q35, Q41

D.1.1 Example 1: Current Smoking Levels

The cross-sectional percentage of young adults who are current smokers reflects both initiation of regular tobacco use and smoking cessation (Table D-2). The age range 18 to 24 years was chosen for the tables in this section because for most people late adolescence and early adulthood are a period of transition. Initiation of regular smoking and development of nicotine addiction occur most often during this age, whereas older adults are less likely to initiate regular tobacco use. Many young adults start smoking as they transition into postsecondary education or full-time employment. Many smokers also quit during this period: national quit rates among smokers in this age group are higher than those among older smokers (USDHHS, 1990).

Table D-2. "Current," "Former," and "Never" Smokers Among All Hispanic Persons Aged 18 to 24, by Country of Birth (Percentage)

	Smoking status		
Country of birth	Current smoker	Former smoker	Never smoker
Mexico			
Central America, South America			
Caribbean			
Spain			
United States			
Other			

Table D-2 shows current smoking prevalence (smoke now, every day, or some days) for Hispanic persons, stratified by country of birth, among persons aged 18 to 24 years. The "smoke now, every day, or some days" question was asked only of respondents who first had indicated that they had smoked at least 100 cigarettes in their lifetime. A "current smoker" is defined, therefore, as a person who has smoked at least 100 cigarettes in his lifetime and was smoking every day or some days at the time of survey. Differences in the initiation of smoking and early adulthood smoking among members of the various racial or ethnic groups seems to be related to numerous variables—sociodemographic, environmental, historical, behavioral, personal, and psychological (USDHHS, 1998).

The adverse health effects of smoking are influenced by both the number of years someone smokes and the intensity of the smoking. The H/L ATS asks about smoking intensity as measured by the number of cigarettes smoked per day (Table D-3). Table D-3 was constructed by recoding Q7 ("About how many cigarettes did you smoke a day . . .") into four categories. The denominator for Table D-3 includes both "every day" and "some days" smokers who reported smoking on at least a single day during the month preceding interview.

Table D-3. Number of Cigarettes Smoked Daily by "Every Day" and "Some Days" Hispanic Smokers Aged 18 to 24, by Country of Birth (Percentage)

	Number of cigarettes smoked daily			
Country of birth	**Less than 1**	**1–10**	**11–20**	**More than 20**
Mexico				
Central America, South America, Caribbean				
Other Latino/Hispanic countries (including Spain)				
United States				
Other				

One good measure of progression to established smoking during adolescence is the cross-sectional prevalence of persons who by early adulthood had smoked at least 100 cigarettes (Table D-4). By "progression to established smoking," we mean that people have advanced through the smoking uptake stages to the point that they are no longer "experimenters" (Mowery, Farrelly, Haviland, Gable, & Wells, 2004).

Table D-4. Whether Hispanic Adults Aged 18 to 24 Smoked 100 Cigarettes in Their Lifetime, by Age (Percentage)

	Smoked 100 cigarettes in lifetime?	
Adult's age	**Yes**	**No**
18–19		
20–24		

Current smoking status among 18- to 19-year-olds reflects the progression to established smoking by age 18 and the incidence of quitting by this age (Table D-5). Because the pattern of initiation and quitting may differ among these groups, Table D-5 is additionally stratified by the self-reported age at which the respondent came to the United States.

Table D-5. "Current," "Former," and "Never Smokers" Among All Hispanic Persons Aged 18 to 19, by Respondent's Age Upon First Entry into the United States (Percentage)

	Smoking status		
Age at first entry into United States	**Never smoker**	**Current smoker**	**Former smoker**
0–11 years			
12–17 years			
18–19 years			

D.1.2 Example 2: Age at Initiation of Smoking

Progression to established smoking depends in part on the age at which people start experimenting with smoking. The H/L ATS asks respondents to report the age at which they first tried a cigarette (Table D-6). A problem with this measure is recall bias because older respondents, especially, may not accurately remember the age at which they first tried a cigarette. Nevertheless, the age of first experimentation with smoking remains an important indicator—one that helps focus interventions on the most appropriate age groups. An important tobacco control strategy has been to try to delay experimentation and regular smoking until late adolescence and early adulthood, a time when most people presumably have better skills and knowledge for rejecting tobacco as an unhealthy practice.

Table D-6. Age at Which Hispanic Persons Aged 30 or Older First Smoked a Cigarette, by Education (Percentage)

	Age first smoked cigarette					
Highest education level completed	**10 or younger**	**11–14**	**15–16**	**17–18**	**19–20**	**21 or older**
Less than high school						
High school graduate						
Some college						
College graduate						

Table D-6 shows the age at which the respondent first tried a cigarette (asked in Q3), by level of education completed, among those who were aged 30 years or older at survey. To make this table, Q3 responses were grouped into age categories. The denominator for Table D-6 includes only those who had ever tried a cigarette (asked in Q2). Level of education is an appropriate domain for this table because most people have completed their formal education by age 30.

Menthol cigarettes are used by some young adults to reduce throat irritation, and some smokers think that menthol cigarettes are less harmful to health than regular cigarettes (Giovino et al., 2004). Table D-7 shows the prevalence of use of menthol cigarettes by

Hispanic young adult current smokers, by whether the respondent thinks that quitting smoking after more than 20 years of smoking will benefit one's health. Analysts may want to be aware that in cognitive testing respondents who answered "No" to the question on whether quitting would benefit health included those who thought the benefits of quitting after smoking so much would be substantial but not great, as well as those who thought there would be no benefits from quitting at that point.

Table D-7. Use of Menthol Cigarettes Among Hispanic Smokers Aged 18 to 24, by Perceived Benefits of Quitting (Percentage)

	Usually smokes menthol cigarettes?	
Thinks quitting smoking after 20+ years will benefit health	**Yes**	**No**
Yes		
No		

D.2 Exposure to Secondhand Smoke

Exposure to secondhand tobacco smoke causes lung cancer, other respiratory diseases, and coronary heart disease in adults; inhalation of tobacco smoke also causes symptoms such as runny nose and throat irritation (USDHHS, 2006). Section D.2 offers some variables for analysis of H/L ATS data on exposure to secondhand smoke. Table D-8 summarizes the variables used in the tables developed to study this topic (Tables D-9 through D-13).

Table D-8. H/L ATS Questions Addressed in Tables D-9 Through D-13

Variable	Table D-9	Table D-10	Table D-11	Table D-12	Table D-13
Outcomes	Q22, Q23, Q25	Q22, Q23, Q24	Q2, Q4, Q5, Q23	Q29, Q30, Q31	Q34a, Q34b, Q34c, Q34d, Q34e, Q40
Domains	Q50	Q4, Q5, Q22, Q23, Q47	Q44	Q26, Q27, Q49a	Q2, Q4, Q5

D.2.1 Example 1: Exposure to Secondhand Smoke at Home

Young children are particularly vulnerable to secondhand smoke in the home because they spend so much time there. Measurement of home exposure to secondhand smoke is accomplished by three means: ambient air monitoring, biological markers of exposure among people who live in the home, and self-reports of exposure. The H/L ATS uses self-report, for which there are two questions: a question about home rules (Q25) and a question about recall of smoking in the home (Q24).

The percentage distribution of restrictions on family members' and guests' smoking in the home is shown in Table D-9. These home rules are stratified by income level, which is recoded into one of four groups from the eight income categories that respondents can self-report (Q50).

Table D-9. Home Smoking Rules Among All Hispanic Adults, by Income (Percentage)

	Smoking permitted inside the home?			
Annual household income ($)	**No, not anywhere or at any time**	**Allowed some places or times**	**Yes, allowed anywhere and at any time**	**Don't know**
Less than 25K				
25K to less than 50K				
50K to less than 75K				
75K or more				

Although home rules can indicate exposure, they do not necessarily measure all secondhand smoke exposure at home, because smoking bans may be ignored. An alternative measure of home exposure among nonsmokers is possible with the H/L ATS: Q24 asks for the number of days that someone, excluding the respondent, smoked in the home during the 7 days preceding interview. Table D-10 shows the percentage of persons who reported that someone other than the respondent smoked in the home during the 7 days preceding the interview, by whether the respondent speaks Spanish or English. Language is being used here as a marker of generation. Usually those who speak English are second or third generation.

Table D-10. Number of Days in Past Week That Someone Smoked Inside Home, by Language Generally Spoken by Adult Respondent (Percentage)

	Number of days smoking occurred in home during last week			
Language spoken	**None**	**1–2**	**3–6**	**7**
Only English, English better than Spanish, or both equally				
Only Spanish or Spanish better than English				

Table D-10 requires some programming to develop. First, one must subset those respondents who are nonsmokers (based on Q4 and Q5). This subset is the denominator. Next, one must recode into appropriate groups the number of days that smoking occurred inside the home. Table D-10 shows only one of the possible recodings. Although it is a valid estimate of the population prevalence of nonsmokers who are exposed to secondhand smoke in their homes, it does not measure the prevalence of households in which people are exposed to secondhand smoke, because the H/L ATS is generally weighted to the population of people, not households. Moreover, Table D-10 does not include home exposure as identified by smoker respondents to the survey.

A measure of children's potential exposure to secondhand smoke is possible with the H/L ATS. Research has shown that the total number of smokers in a household is correlated with increased serum cotinine levels—more so than number of days someone smoked in the home is correlated (Pirkle et al., 1996). Combining Q5 (whether respondent is a smoker) and Q23 (smoking status of all other adults in the home, excluding the respondent) yields the number of smokers in the household. Table D-11 shows the percentage of respondents who live in homes with one or more smokers, by the age of children in the home. Note that the outcome for Table D-11 (number of smokers in the home) does not include adolescent smokers. Also note that the domain levels in Table D-11 are not mutually exclusive. For example, a respondent who lives in a home with a newborn and a 5-year-old child will be counted in two rows of the table.

Table D-11. Number of Smokers in Home, by Age of Children in Home (Percentage)

	Number of smokers in home			
Age of children in home	**None**	**1**	**2**	**More than 2**
Newborn to 11 months old				
1–4 years old				
5–11 years old				
12–17 years old				

Because parents may choose not to smoke at home when their children are present, a smoker in the home with children is a good indicator of children's potential exposure but not as good a measure of actual exposure. Smoking at any time in the home may expose children later, however, because secondhand smoke tar is deposited on surfaces and evaporates as fine particles (Nazaroff & Singer, 2004). The levels of delayed exposure and risk from this exposure are as yet unknown.

D.2.2 Example 2: Exposure of Nonsmokers to Workplace Secondhand Smoke

The H/L ATS asks about workplace smoking policy that applies to the respondent's work areas (Q30) and indoor worksite public areas (Q31). Another indicator of exposure to secondhand smoke is Q28, which asks respondents whether they recall anyone's smoking in their work area in the week preceding the survey. These questions are asked only of respondents who are employed for wages or who are self-employed and work outside the home. Table D-12 shows the prevalence of workplace smoking policies by education level. Table D-12 was constructed as a recode of Q30 and Q31.

Table D-12. Workplace Smoking Policy for Indoor Work Areas and Indoor Public Areas Used by Hispanic Nonsmoking Workers, by Education (Percentage)

	Workplace smoking policy for indoor work areas and indoor public areas				
Highest education level completed	**Smoking not allowed in any work or public area**	**Smoking prohibited in some or all work areas only**	**Smoking prohibited in some or all public areas only**	**Smoking allowed in work and public areas**	**No official rule**
Less than high school					
High school graduate					
Some college					
College graduate					

D.2.3 Example 3: Attitudes Toward Laws on Clean Indoor Air

Through ordinances and regulations, state and local governments can mandate that nonsmokers be protected from secondhand smoke in public places. Public support for banning smoking in public places increased dramatically during the past 20 years. As of 2001, about 1,200 local ordinances restricting smoking in public places had been enacted (Brownson, Hopkins, & Wakefield, 2002). In addition, many states, including Arizona, California, and Massachusetts, have enacted comprehensive bans on smoking in public indoor places—for example, bans in workplaces, restaurants, and bars (ANRF, 2007).

The H/L ATS contains a set of questions that measure respondents' support for smoking bans in indoor places. There are five questions (Q34a, Q34b, Q34c, Q34d, Q34d), each asking about a different venue. In addition, Q40a measures support for clean indoor air in a different way by asking whether the respondent would support a smoking ban in most indoor places but excluding bars, night clubs, and casinos. Table D-13 can be used to assess public support for smoking bans and to determine possible barriers to the enactment of a 100% ban.

Table D-13 was constructed by appending six separate cross-tabulations, one for each question. Standard statistical analyses like chi-square tests cannot be performed with this data structure that allows each respondent to be represented multiple times. It is possible to test for a difference in attitudes between one status and all others. For statistical methods for comparing two binomial proportions, see Fleiss, Levin, and Paik (2003). Table D-13 is stratified by respondent smoking status.

Table D-13. Whether Hispanic Adult Respondents Think Smoking Should Be Prohibited in Worksites and Other Indoor Places, by Smoking Status (Percentage)

	Thinks smoking should be prohibited in all areas of					
Smoking status	**Public places (government buildings, banks, malls)**	**Work places**	**Restaurants**	**Bars, taverns, night clubs**	**Casinos**	**Supports law banning smoking in other places**
Current smoker						
Former smoker						
Never smoker						

D.3 Smoking Cessation

Information about smoking cessation is important to the crafting of intervention programs. Section D.3 offers some variables for analysis of H/L ATS data on smoking cessation. Table D-14 summarizes the variables used in the analyses (Tables D-15, D-16, and D-17).

Table D-14. H/L ATS Questions Addressed in Tables D-15 Through D-17

Variable	Table D-15	Table D-16	Table D-17
Outcomes	Q12, Q15, Q16	Q13, Q14, Q21, Q21a	Q11
Domains	Q2, Q4, Q5, Q53	Q2, Q4, Q5, Q42	Q2, Q4, Q5

D.3.1 Example 1: Stages of Change

The H/L ATS can be used to develop an index for the prevalence of smokers who are ready to quit smoking (Table D-15). The stage-of-change index shown in Table D-15 is based on a series of questions, including whether the respondent had made a quit attempt during the 12 months preceding the survey (Q12); readiness to quit in the next 6 months (Q15); and readiness to quit in the next 30 days (Q16).

Respondents who at the time of interview were not seriously considering quitting in the next 6 months are "precontemplators." Those who were seriously considering quitting in the next 6 months but not in the next 30 days are "contemplators." Those who were planning to quit in the next 30 days but who had not made a serious quit attempt in the past year are in the "preparation" stage. Those smokers who were planning to quit in the next 30 days and who had made a quit attempt in the past year are in the "action" stage. The stage-of-change index is constructed only for current smokers.

Table D-15. Hispanic Current Smokers' Stage of Change Toward Smoking Cessation, by Whether Spouse or Partner Uses Tobacco (Percentage)

Spouse or partner currently smokes or uses smokeless tobacco?	Stage of change toward smoking cessation			
	Precontemplation	Contemplation	Preparation	Action
Yes				
No				

The delineation of stages of change in Table D-15 is not universally used. Moreover, the stage of change can measure only readiness to quit and cannot be used to infer actual quit attempts or success in quitting: quit attempts can be triggered by environmental changes; success in quitting depends on a host of other factors, including degree of addiction, level of self-efficacy for quitting, and level of self-confidence for quitting.

D.3.2 Example 2: Methods Used to Quit at Last Quit Attempt

Many therapies, self-help materials, and programs have been developed to assist individuals in quitting smoking. On the H/L ATS, three assisted-quitting methods were asked about independently; respondents could choose more than one method. Use of medications, including nicotine replacement therapy, is asked about in Q13. Q14 asks about the use of classes or counseling. Q21 and Q21a ask about seeking help in quitting from other persons, such as a medicine man, herbalist, or religious leader. Cessation method questions are asked of both current and former smokers.

Table D-16 shows the prevalence of use of the three assisted-quitting methods. Nicotine replacement therapy and classes or counseling reference the last quit attempt, whereas seeking help from other persons references a 12-month recall period. It is possible to test for a difference in prevalence of use between males and females. For statistical methods for comparing two binomial proportions, see Fleiss, Levin, and Paik (2003).

Table D-16. Methods Used to Quit Smoking Among Hispanic Current and Former Smokers, by Gender (Percentage)

	Method used for last quit attempt		Consulted in past 12 months
Gender	Nicotine patch, nicotine gum, or other medication	Classes or counseling	Saw a medicine man, santero, spiritist, herbalist, religious leader, or other non–health professional
Male			
Female			

D.3.3 Example 3: Length of Abstinence Among Former Smokers

Smokers and ex-smokers typically report making multiple attempts to quit (USDHHS, 1990). Among those who have quit for a single day, the failure rate is very high. The longer the quit attempt lasts, the more likely it is that the individual will successfully avoid relapsing. The length of abstinence is used as an indicator of smokers' overall success in quitting and an indirect measure of smokers' knowledge of resources to help them quit. Table D-17 shows the length of abstinence for former smokers. The outcome variable for Table D-17 is a recode of Q11. The denominator for this table is persons who had smoked at least 100 cigarettes in their lifetime but were not smoking at time of interview (ascertained from Q2, Q4, and Q5). Respondents who reported in Q11 that they never smoked regularly are excluded from the denominator.

Table D-17. Length of Abstinence Among Hispanic Current and Former Smokers, by Age (Percentage)

	Length of abstinence			
Age	**Up to 1 month**	**1–3 months**	**3 months to 1 year**	**Longer than 1 year**
18–24 years				
25–44 years				
45–64 years				
65 years or older				

D.4 Use of Additional Data Sets

Reviewing findings from other reputable tobacco-related studies and relating that information to the target population can expand one's perspective, providing a fuller understanding of tobacco-related issues as they affect that specific population. Section D.4 presents two such analyses.

Table D-18 summarizes the H/L ATS variables used in the comparison presented in Table D-20 (no H/L ATS findings are presented in Table D-19).

Table D-18. H/L ATS Question Addressed in Tables D-19 and D-20

Variable	Table D-19	Table D-20
Outcomes	TUS-CPS	Q36
Domains	TUS-CPS	ANRF

D.4.1 Example 1: Occupational Differences in Workplace Smoking Policies

Table D-12 shows workplace smoking policies by education level, based on the H/L ATS. We can further explore differences in workplace policies among population groups by using the Tobacco Use Supplement (TUS) to the Current Population Survey (CPS). The TUS-CPS is a national survey that is prestratified by state (i.e., the sample is drawn independently within each state). There are enough completed interviews at the state level to make reliable individual state estimates for many domains. A rich set of respondent and household occupational information is made available by linking responses to the TUS with items collected through the CPS. For example, Table D-19 shows workplace smoking polices by three broad occupational categories: white collar, blue collar, and food service. Although many business organizations have adopted smoke-free worksite policies, certain industries lag behind, particularly food service establishments and bars that serve the public (Shopland, Anderson, Burns, & Gerlach, 2004). Servers and other food service workers are often exposed to secondhand tobacco smoke while working. The occupational categories shown in Table D-19 are a recode based on the detailed occupational codes used by the CPS (U.S. Census Bureau, 2006). The TUS-CPS is sponsored by the National Cancer Institute and is fielded every 3 years.

Table D-19. U.S. Employed Smokers[a] Who Work in Smoke-free, Smoking-allowed, and No-policy Workplaces, by Occupation (Percentage)[b,c]

	Workplace smoking policy		
Occupation class	**No policy**	**Smoking allowed**	**Smoke-free**
White collar			
Blue collar			
Food service			

[a]Respondents who reported smoking every day one year prior to survey.

[b]Table excludes self-employed persons and persons who work outdoors.

[c]Source: 2001–2002 NCI Tobacco Use Supplement to the Current Population Survey.

D.4.2 Example 2: Merging H/L ATS Data with Environmental Data

The H/L ATS can be used to assess differences in attitudes and beliefs about exposure to secondhand smoke and to determine whether the respondent lives in a locality with a law on clean indoor air. Q36 asks respondents whether they think that breathing secondhand smoke is harmful to one's health. This question is the outcome for Table D-20.

Table D-20. Beliefs About the Harmful Effects of Breathing Secondhand Smoke, by Strength of Local Clean Indoor Air Laws (Percentage)

	Belief About breathing secondhand smoke		
Strength of local law on clean indoor air	**Harmful to one's health**	**Not harmful at all to one's health**	**Don't know**
100% ban[a]			
Qualified[b]			
Weak or no law			

[a]Law prohibits smoking in all worksites and all public indoor places, including restaurants and freestanding bars.

[b]Law allows exemptions for some indoor places.

Information on the domain for Table D-20, the strength of local laws mandating clean indoor air, is available from the Americans for Nonsmokers' Rights Foundation (ANRF; http://no-smoke.org/). Since 1985 ANRF has tracked, collected, and analyzed local tobacco control ordinances, bylaws, and Board of Health regulations (ANRF, 2007). As of January 3, 2006, the database contained more than 5,000 ordinances from more than 2,900 communities. Each ordinance database record has more than 200 fields detailing characteristics of the law or regulation for each municipality. Table D-20 uses one of the primary fields in the ANRF database: whether the local ordinance completely bans smoking in public indoor places, whether the local ordinance is qualified (meaning that the ordinance exempts certain indoor places), or whether the local ordinance is weak or there is no local ordinance for clean indoor air. Information on the strength of local laws can be merged to the H/L ATS by zip code (Q55). Information on local ordinances for a specific state can be obtained by contractual agreement with ANRF.

E. ENHANCING RESPONSE RATES

Survey researchers are well aware of the importance of achieving the high response rates critical to establishing the reliability and accuracy of survey findings. There are many well-known methods for doing so (AAPOR, 2006). In this section, in order to distill lessons specific to improving response rates for the Hispanic/Latino Adult Tobacco Survey (H/L ATS), we focus on the experience of researchers who have surveyed Hispanic and Latino populations.

Overall Comments

First, there are no "silver bullet" solutions to the problem of raising survey response rates. Survey response rates have consistently declined over the past 20 years across all segments of the population. Second, much of the evidence concerning specific recommendations for enhancing response rates among Hispanic and Latino populations is anecdotal. Usually the race or ethnicity of the nonrespondents is unknown, precluding rigorous quantitative analysis. What is known about effective techniques is often based on qualitative review of call history records and interviewers' impressions of the relative success they have using different approaches.

Using the H/L ATS

Seasoned survey researchers generally affirm that using approaches sensitive to the specific cultural and social context of the target population will help achieve the highest rates possible. The foremost method we can recommend for improving response rates among the Hispanic/Latino population is, therefore, the use of the H/L ATS itself. As described in Section F.1, the survey design and the questionnaire were carefully developed to be sensitive to the specific cultural and social contexts of Hispanic and Latino populations in the United States. The better the respondents can relate to the survey—the introduction, the questions, their communications with the interviewer—the more likely they are to cooperate and complete the interview.

Advance Letters

Advance letters generally aid in increasing survey participation and in reducing the number of contacts required to obtain a full response to the survey (Dillman, 2000). Anecdotal findings reported by Schoua-Glusberg (1998, 2000) affirm the value of advance letters in helping win respondent cooperation. Section B.5 details how the H/L ATS advance letter can be incorporated into the survey protocol.

Customized Introductions

Experienced survey researchers understand the importance of an effective introduction to create rapport with respondents and to gain their cooperation. A researcher experienced in surveying Hispanic/Latino populations offered CDC the following advice on developing effective introductions with Hispanic/Latino persons:

> Many [Hispanic/Latino] people do not really understand what surveys are for and how health-related surveys are the source of the data that serve not only for planning, but also for better educating the community. We understand that IRB [institutional review board] issues require significant formality, but a brief explanation of what the survey is and what the information will serve for early in the introduction tends to boost participation. . . .
>
> We also found that the straightforward and somewhat cold presentation of the survey when the first person answers the phone increases the nonparticipation rates. The presentation of the survey needs to be friendlier and with opportunities to ask feedback from the person who answers the call. . . .
>
> We found that "asking for a favor" is key. . . . When we tell them that we are asking a favor from them, they understand right away the social value of the survey. (Personal communication, June 7, 2006)

Appropriate Response to Concerns

The success of a good interviewer often rests in his or her ability to quickly perceive and respond to the concerns of potential respondents. It is worthwhile for researchers administering the H/L ATS to invest in developing effective responses to frequently asked questions and in training interviewers to use those answers. This correspondence with CDC specifies, "It is also very important to clarify that it is not about selling anything to them, or that it is not at all a market-related call." The report issued after CDC's 2002 expert meeting, *Effective Tobacco Control in Hispanic/Latino Communities: A Synopsis of Key Findings and Recommendations* (USDHHS, 2004), provides insight into ways to approach Hispanic and Latino persons and the concerns they have about participating in surveys.

Bilingual Interviewers

The H/L ATS is available in Spanish, and use of the Spanish version will help ensure that bias is not introduced by way of failure to interview monolingual Spanish speakers. Beyond this measure, however, interviewers should be able to alternate easily between English and Spanish during the initial contact with a household. Even if some household members speak English, some members, particularly older members or recent immigrants, may speak only Spanish. It is most efficient for the interviewer to be able to immediately conduct the introduction and screener with the person who answers the phone, whether that person speaks English or speaks Spanish. Even when the screener or interview is conducted in English, it may be helpful for the interviewer to be able to answer respondents' questions in Spanish. For maximum flexibility and response rate, therefore, we recommend that all interviewers be bilingual and that they be assessed for their bilingual skill before being allowed on the telephone.

F. BACKGROUND, REFERENCES, AND RESOURCES

This guide is intended to be used by health practitioners, researchers, and statisticians who are interested in collecting data on tobacco use, cessation, secondhand smoke, risk perceptions and social influences, and demographic information from Hispanic/Latino populations. Specific sections of the guide may be most appropriate for specific uses: health practitioners might use Sections A, B, and F; interviewer training may benefit most from Section B; and researchers and statisticians may want to consult Sections C, D, and E. In this section we provide this array of users with the detailed history, theoretical demands, and practical considerations informing the Hispanic/Latino Adult Tobacco Survey (H/L ATS). We conclude with a bibliographic list of resources subdivided by content area of the guide. Contact information completes the resources offered here.

F.1 Background to the Development of the H/L ATS

The H/L ATS is a culturally appropriate adult tobacco use questionnaire administered to determine among Hispanic and Latino adults in the United States the prevalence of tobacco use, exposure to secondhand smoke, and exposure to influences for and against tobacco use. The availability of a consistent, well-developed questionnaire will improve the quality of this information, which will in turn aid in the development of culturally sensitive and effective tobacco control programs for Hispanic and Latino populations. Section F.1 provides the user of this guide with the background and rationale for the development of these survey materials.

F.1.1 Purpose of a Culturally Appropriate H/L ATS

Hispanic and Latino persons residing in the United States embody a unique set of attitudes, behaviors, knowledge, experience, and other cultural characteristics. These characteristics call for a customized approach to measuring health-compromising behaviors such as tobacco use, in order that truly effective cessation and prevention programs may be developed in this population at the local, state, and regional levels (Kerner, Breen, Tefft, & Silsby, 1998). To this end, in 2002, under the direction of the Centers for Disease Control and Prevention (CDC), Office on Smoking and Health (OSH), the General Population State ATS was adapted to create the H/L ATS. The H/L ATS was designed specifically to measure general health, tobacco use, cessation, exposure to secondhand smoke, risk perceptions, social influences, and demographics among Hispanic and Latino adults.

For information and background on the General Population State ATS, see the *Guidelines for Conducting General Population State Adult Tobacco Surveys* (Mariolis, in press).

Growth in Hispanic and Latino Populations

The need for targeted, culturally sensitive tobacco use prevention programs is substantiated by the growing number of Hispanic and Latino persons residing in the United States. The

U.S. Hispanic and Latino population already constitutes a large portion of the overall population, and the numbers are increasing rapidly. According to the U.S. Census Bureau, in 2003 there were 39.9 million Hispanic/Latino persons living in the United States (U.S. Census Bureau, 2004), a 78% increase over 1990 (22.4 million). It is expected that the number of Hispanic/Latino persons living in the United States will increase to 102.6 million by the year 2050. If these Census projections are correct, 24.4%, or about 1 of every 4 persons residing in the United States, will be of Hispanic or Latino origin (U.S. Census Bureau, 2004).

If the Hispanic/Latino adult smoking prevalence remains at its average level of 18.3% (1990–1999) for the next 50 years, the number of Hispanic and Latino adult smokers will increase from 3.8 million in the year 2000 to 11.0 million in the year 2050. Although the H/L ATS is not administered to those under the age of 18, data on adults will inform prevention programs for younger Hispanic and Latino persons, who are the largest minority youth population in the United States and 16% of the population under age 18 (Flores et al., 2002).

Tobacco Use and Exposure Among Hispanic and Latino Populations

The Hispanic and Latino populations in the United States face unique challenges that put them at higher risk than the general population for tobacco use and exposure to smoke:

- Depending on location, about one fifth of Hispanic or Latino persons have low English-language skills (U.S. Census Bureau, 2004).
- The Hispanic and Latino populations are likely to have limited exposure to anti–tobacco use information, educational materials, media messages, and cessation services, compared with those who have better English-language skills.
- The Hispanic and Latino populations continue to be the target of intensive tobacco-industry marketing efforts. These efforts include sponsorship of cultural events, funding of Hispanic and Latino organizations and issues, and other targeted marketing efforts.
- Initial evidence suggests that Hispanic and Latino workers tend to be more exposed than other workers to secondhand smoke on the job. This increased exposure occurs even though Hispanic and Latino populations often demonstrate high levels of awareness of the health risks posed by secondhand smoke, as well as strong support for smoke-free policies.
- As Hispanic and Latino persons become more acculturated, initial findings suggest that their rate of smoking is increasing and approaching that of the general population. This trend is of particular concern with regard to younger people.

Several issues pertain directly to the design and implementation of successful tobacco control programs in the Hispanic and Latino population assessed with the H/L ATS:

- Prevalence of "occasional," or nondaily, smoking.
- Increase in use of menthol cigarettes.
- Prevalence of smoking cessation and quit attempts.

- Methods used to quit, including nontraditional methods possibly unique to Hispanic/Latino persons.
- Rules and perceptions about secondhand smoke exposure in the home and at work.
- Additional demographic considerations (e.g., country of birth, education and income levels, length of stay in the United States).

Hispanic and Latino communities have unique strengths and assets conducive to effective tobacco control initiatives. By acting now to help these communities implement sustained, culturally appropriate tobacco control interventions, researchers and health practitioners can avert the predicted rise in smoking and the associated danger of smoking-related disease.

F.1.2 Design of the H/L ATS Questionnaires and Survey Methodology

CDC convened a meeting of leading researchers and health program administrators, "Effective Tobacco Control in Hispanic/Latino Communities," in August 2002. The purpose of this meeting was to address questions about tobacco control specifically as it relates to program, policy, communication, surveillance, and evaluation in various Hispanic and Latino populations. The subsequent findings and recommendations specific to surveillance needs assisted in the development of the H/L ATS. Recommendations that directly influenced the development of the H/L ATS included the following:

- Increase sample sizes to generate more precise estimates of tobacco use prevalence in Hispanic and Latino populations.
- Collect information on secondhand smoke exposure rates and on attitudes toward public policy.
- Appropriately adapt, both culturally and linguistically, survey questions for the Hispanic/Latino population.
- Monitor the prevalence of and trends in "occasional smoking" among Hispanic and Latino populations.
- Collect data at the regional and state levels.
- Track and analyze the effects of acculturation, income levels, and education levels on tobacco use prevalence and behaviors among Hispanic and Latino populations.
- Conduct research on whether differences in tobacco use prevalence between specific Hispanic/Latino populations are due to differences in culture or to differences in class and income (or socioeconomic) status.
- Examine the reasons for disparities among various Hispanic/Latino populations.

During the meeting, strong consensus emerged that tobacco control interventions that acknowledge and highlight the cultural strengths, assets, and protective factors of the Hispanic and Latino population would be most effective. Conversely, it was agreed that interventions that failed to recognize the unique linguistic, social, and cultural characteristics of this population would be relatively ineffective.

Questionnaire Design

During the August 2002 meeting, 10 researchers reviewed the OSH General Population State Adult Tobacco Telephone Survey. These 10 researchers were selected for the review of the survey instrument because of their expertise in tobacco control and their research experience with specific Hispanic and Latino subpopulations (e.g., Mexican American, Puerto Rican, and Cuban). The researchers advised OSH which questions were appropriate and which were inappropriate for Hispanic and Latino populations.

Five of the original 10 researchers were subsequently identified to provide more in-depth recommendations on how to adapt the survey for the Hispanic and Latino population. A second meeting was held at CDC, where the five researchers and an OSH epidemiologist continued to modify the General Population State ATS to make the questions more culturally appropriate for Hispanic and Latino subgroups. In addition, new questions specific to Hispanic and Latino populations were added to the instrument, such as the following: "In the past 12 months, have you seen a medicine man (curandero), santero, spiritist (espiritista), herbalist (yerbero), religious leaders (priest, pastor, rabbi, etc.), or other non-health professionals to help you quit smoking?" New demographic questions also elicit country of birth, educational levels, income levels, and language preference.

Survey Methodology

The H/L ATS is meant to be readily usable by public health organizations at all levels. The H/L ATS can be administered either as a telephone interview or as an in-person interview, and in English or Spanish.[7] Two of the case studies described in Section C use telephone administration, and the third uses in-person interviewing. Each of the case studies selected the administration mode that best suited its particular study population. To further increase the usability of the H/L ATS, complementary survey materials (i.e., screeners, consent forms, and advance letters in both English and Spanish) were developed as part of the H/L ATS package.[8] All materials are publicly available to jurisdictions, organizations, and individuals.

F.1.3 Development of Spanish Versions of the H/L ATS

Consensus Approach to Translation

Committee approaches to translation have been used since the 1960s (Nida, 1964) and more recently in the translation of data collection instruments (Acquadro, Jambon, Ellis, &

[7] The H/L ATS questionnaire and screener are available in three versions: all English, all Spanish, and Spanish with English instructions for interviewers and programmers. The designers of the H/L ATS have anticipated that the survey may be used in countries where Spanish is the national language. The "all Spanish" version is appropriate when all interviewers, programmers, and survey staff are Spanish monolinguals. The "Spanish with English instructions" version is appropriate when it is expected that those programming the computerized version of the questionnaire will be English monolinquals.

[8] The consent form and consent text provided here differ slightly from those used in CDC's 2007 survey.

Marquis, 1996; Brislin, 1976; Guillemin, Bombardier, & Beaton, 1993; Schoua-Glusberg, 1992). Moreover, the Census Bureau guideline for survey translation now recommends this approach (U.S. Census Bureau, 2004). Its strength is that consensus among bilinguals produces more accurate text than the subjective opinion of a single translator: problems of personal idiosyncrasies, culture, and uneven skill in either language are overcome. Translation by committee produced the Spanish version of the H/L ATS.

The core modules of the H/L ATS were originally translated into Spanish by an epidemiologist within OSH. This translation underwent review by a team of three translators who are native speakers of some of the main varieties of Spanish spoken in the United States (Mexican, Puerto Rican, and South American). This review was refereed by a specialist with 2 decades of experience in chairing survey translation committees. For the supplemental modules, there existed no original Spanish translation. The team of three translators worked independently, translating from English one third of the protocol each. After this initial translation, another refereed reconciliation meeting was held to ensure each item reflected the intent of the English original and was equally effective in Spanish.

In reconciliation meetings, each translator contributed to the discussion to improve and refine the translation, in order to make the Spanish culturally appropriate for the three majority Latino or Hispanic populations. In the discussions, each member was required to articulate the reasons for suggested changes or improvements to the original translation. The team looked together for alternative translations, finally selecting by consensus.

Cognitive Research to Enhance Cultural Adaptation

Upon completion of the translations, the questionnaires were subjected to extensive cognitive testing with members of the target populations residing in Miami, New York City, El Paso, and Chicago. Cognitive testing was conducted to establish that the questions are culturally appropriate and sensible; that they will be understood similarly across participants of different national origins, education levels, or income levels; and that the Spanish translation works well across such a diversity of respondents. As is the case in every cognitive evaluation project, a goal was also to identify any question-processing problems or difficulties respondents might experience—including cognitive complexity of questions, words not understood, problems in stems or response categories, and recall issues—that could lead to measurement error.

Cognitive interviews are a qualitative method that determines not only which items work and which present problems, but also *why* certain items do not work. Because they are bilingual, translators are systematically different from the monolingual (and often monocultural) population for whom the translated instrument is prepared. With the use of such qualitative methods, the generation of a translated text brings together, at each stage of the process, the combined efforts of professional translators and the input of the audience.

Sixty-eight interviews—19 in English, and 49 in Spanish—were conducted in two rounds, between June 2004 and April 2005 (Table F-1). Recruiting for interviews was accomplished through community organizations and agencies in each city.

Table F-1. National Origin, City of Residence, and Language of Interview for Respondents to the H/L ATS Cognitive Testing

Origin and residence	Spanish interviews	English interviews
Mexico		
Chicago	2	0
El Paso	12	0
Puerto Rico		
Chicago	3	1
New York	5	3
Cuba		
Chicago	1	0
Miami	5	5
El Salvador		
Chicago	3	0
Columbia		
Chicago	4	0
Dominican Republic		
Chicago	2	0
New York	5	5
Guatemala		
Chicago	4	1
Ecuador		
Chicago	0	2
Honduras		
Chicago	1	2
Peru		
Chicago	2	0

Findings from the first round of interviews were used to make changes intended to reduce or eliminate problems and error. In the second round, these changes were tested. The current, final version of the English and Spanish H/L ATS includes the modifications stemming from both rounds of cognitive interviews. The resulting version is suitable for the broader Latino population of the United States.

F.2 References and Resources

F.2.1 Background to Hispanic/Latino Surveying and the ATS

Flores G, Fuentes-Afflick E, Barbot O, Carter-Pokras O, Claudio L, Lara M, et al. The health of Latino children: urgent priorities, unanswered questions, and a research agenda. *Journal of the American Medical Association* 2002;288(1):82–90.

Kerner J, Breen N, Tefft M, Silsby J. Tobacco use among multi-ethnic Latino populations. *Ethnicity & Disease* 1998;8(2):167–183.

Mariolis M. *Guidelines for Conducting General Population State Adult Tobacco Surveys.* Atlanta, GA: U.S. Department of Health and Human Services, Centers for Disease Control and Prevention; in press.

U.S. Census Bureau. *U.S. Census Report: Language Use and English Speaking Ability.* Available at http://www.census.gov/prod/2003pubs/c2kbr-29.pdf.

Waksberg J, Levine D, Marker D. *Assessment of Major Federal Data Sets for Analyses of Hispanic and Asian or Pacific Islander Subgroups and Native Americans: Extending the Utility of Federal Data Bases.* Washington, DC: U.S. Department of Health and Human Services, Office of the Assistant Secretary for Planning and Evaluation; 2000. Available at http://aspe.hhs.gov/hsp/minority-db00/task3/section2.htm.

F.2.2 Instrumentation

Acquadro C, Jambon B, Ellis D, Marquis P. Language and translation issues. In: Spilker B, editor. *Quality Life and Pharmacoeconomics in Clinical Trials.* 2nd edition. Philadelphia: Lippincott-Raven; 1996:575–585.

Al-Tayyib AA, Rogers SM, Gribble JN, Villarroel M, Turner CF. Effect of low medical literacy on health survey measurements. *American Journal of Public Health* 2002:92;1478–1481.

Bernal H, Wooley S, Schensul JJ. The challenge of using Likert-type scales with low-literate ethnic populations. *Nursing Research* 1997;46:179–181.

Brislin R. Introduction. In: Brislin R, editor. *Translation: Applications and Research*. New York: Gardner; 1976.

Brodie M, Steffenson A, Valdez J, Levin R, Suro R. *2002 National Survey of Latinos.* Menlo Park, CA: Henry J. Kaiser Family Foundation; 2002. Washington, DC: Pew Hispanic Center. Available at http://www.kff.org/kaiserpolls/20021217a-index.cfm.

Carley-Baxter L, Link MW, Roe D, Quiroz RS. Does context really matter? Results from a Spanish language advance letter pilot. Presentation to the American Association for Public Opinion Research (AAPOR) conference, Montreal, Canada, May 2006.

Dillman DA. *Mail and Internet Surveys: The Tailored Design Method.* New York: Wiley; 2000.

Dillman DA, Redline C, Carley-Baxter L. Influence of type of question on skip pattern compliance in self-administered questionnaires. *Proceedings of the American Statistical Association, Section on Survey Methods.* 2000.

Erkut S, Alarcon O, Garcia CC, Tropp LR, Vazquez Garcia HA. The "dual focus" approach to creating bilingual measures. *Journal of Cross-Cultural Psychology* 1999;30:206–218.

Gallagher PM, Fowler FJ, Stringfellow VL. Hablamos español: collecting information by mail from Spanish-speaking Medicaid enrollees. Paper presented to the American Association of Public Opinion Research (AAPOR) conference, St. Petersburg Beach, FL, May 1999.

Guillemin F, Bombardier C, Beaton D. Cross-cultural adaptation of health-related quality of life measures: literature review and proposed guidelines. *Journal of Clinical Epidemiology* 1993;46:1417–1432.

Harris-Kojetin LD, Fowler FJ, Brown JA, Schnaier JA, Sweeny SF. The use of cognitive testing to develop and evaluate CAHPS 1.0 core survey items. *Medical Care* 1999;37:MS10–MS21.

Herdman M, Fox-Rushby J, Badia X. "Equivalence" and the translation and adaptation of health-related quality of life questionnaires. *Quality of Life Research* 1997;6:237–247.

Marin G, Marin BVO. Research with Hispanic populations. *Applied Social Research Methods Series* 1991;23:1–130.

McKay RB, Breslow MJ, Sangster RL, Gabbard SM, Reynolds RW, Nakamoto JM, et al. Translating survey questionnaires: lessons learned. *New Directions in Evaluation* 1996;70:93–104.

Morales LS, Weidmer BO, Hays RD. Readability of CAHPS 2.0 Child and Adult Core Surveys. In: M. Cynamon M, Kulka R, editors. *Seventh Conference on Health Survey Research Methods.* Hyattsville, MD: U.S. Department of Health and Human Services; 2001:83–90.

Nida EA. *Toward a Science of Translating*. Leiden, Netherlands: Brill; 1964.

Rosal MC, Carbone ET, Goins KV. Use of cognitive interviewing to adapt measurement instruments for low-literate Hispanics. *Diabetes Educator* 2003;29:1006–1017.

Schoua-Glusberg A. *Report on the Translation of the Questionnaire for the National Treatment Improvement Evaluation Study.* Chicago: National Opinion Research Center; 1992.

Schoua-Glusberg A. Screening households in Chicago: Latino cooperation rate in the Project on Human Development in Chicago Neighborhoods (PHDCN). Poster session presented at Hearing the Unheard: Interviewing Minorities, University of Nebraska Survey Research Center 2nd Annual Symposium, Lincoln, April 1998.

Schoua-Glusberg A. *Privacy, Census and Surveys: Latinos' Views: Final Report for Protecting Privacy Project Contract Research.* Washington, DC: U.S. Department of Commerce, Census Bureau; 2000.

U.S. Census Bureau. *Census Bureau Guideline: Language Translation of Data Collection Instruments and Supporting Materials.* Washington, DC: U.S. Department of Commerce, Census Bureau; 2004. Available at http://www.census.gov/cac/www/007585.html.

Weech-Maldonado R, Weidmer BO, Morales LS, Hays RD. Cross-cultural adaptation of survey instruments: the CAHPS experience. In: *Seventh Conference on Health Survey Research Methods*. Hyattsville, MD: U.S. Department of Health and Human Services, Centers for Disease Control and Prevention; 2000:75–82. Available at http://www.cdc.gov/nchs/data/conf/conf07.pdf.

F.2.3 Sampling and Weighting

Albright V, DiSogra C, Krotki K, Bye L. Special challenges of conducting research in California. Presentation to the annual meeting of the Society for Applied Sociology, Sacramento, CA, October 2002.

American Association of Public Opinion Research (AAPOR). *Standard Definitions: Final Dispositions of Case Codes and Outcome Rates for Surveys.* Lenexa, KS: AAPOR; 2004.

Biernacki P, Waldorf D. Snowball sampling: problems and techniques of chain referral sampling. *Sociological Methods and Research* 1981;10(2):141–163.

Birnbaum ZW, Sirken MG. *Design of Sample Surveys to Estimate the Prevalence of Rare Diseases: Three Unbiased Estimates.* Series 2, No. 11. U.S. Department of Health and Human Services, Centers for Disease Control and Prevention, National Center for Health Statistics, Vital and Health Statistics. Washington, DC: U.S. Government Printing Office; 1965.

Blair J, Czaja R. Locating a special population using random digit dialing. *Public Opinion Quarterly* 1982;46(4):585–590.

Blumberg SJ, Halfon N, Olson LM. The national survey of early childhood health. *Pediatrics* 2004;113:1899–1906.

Boyle WR, Kalsbeek WD. Extensions to the two-stratum model for sampling rare subgroups in telephone surveys. *Proceedings of the Section on Survey Research Methods, American Statistical Association*. 2005. [CD-ROM].

Carr K, HertvikJ. Within-household selection: is anybody listening? *Proceedings of the Section on Survey Research Methods, American Statistical Association.* 1993:1119–1123.

Casady RJ, Lepkowski JM. Optimal allocation for stratified telephone survey designs. *Proceedings of the Section on Survey Research Methods, American Statistical Association.* 1991:111–116.

Casady RJ, Lepkowski JM. Stratified telephone survey designs. *Survey Methodology* 1993;19:103–113.

Cochran WG. *Sampling Techniques.* 3rd edition. New York: Wiley; 1977.

Deville JC, Särndal CE. Calibration estimators in survey sampling. *Journal of the American Statistical Association* 1992;87:376–382.

Gaziano C. Comparative analysis of within-household respondent selection techniques. *Public Opinion Quarterly* 2005;69(1):124–157.

Hartley HO. Multiple frame methodology and selected applications. *Sankhya: The Indian Journal of Statistics* 1974;36C:99–118.

Horvitz DG, Thompson DJ. A generalization of sampling without replacement from a finite universe. *Journal of the American Statistical Association* 1952;47:663–685.

Iannacchione VG, Staab JM, Redden DT. Evaluating the use of residential mailing addresses in a metropolitan household survey. *Proceedings of the Section on Survey Research Methods, American Statistical Association.* 2003:4028–4033.

Johnson RL, Saha S, Arbelaez JJ, Beach MC, Cooper LA. Racial and ethnic differences in patient perceptions of bias and cultural competence in health care. *Journal of General Internal Medicine* 2004;19(2):101–110.

Kalsbeek WD. Sampling minority groups in health surveys. *Statistics in Medicine* 2003;22:1527–1549.

Kalsbeek WD, Agans RP. Sampling and weighting in household telephone surveys. In: Lepkowski JM, et al., editors. *Advances in Telephone Survey Methodology.* New York: Wiley; 2007.

Kalsbeek WD, Boyle WR, Agans RP, White JE. Disproportionate sampling for population subgroups in telephone surveys. *Statistics in Medicine* 2007;26(8):1657–1674.

Kalsbeek WD, Kavanagh ST, Wu J. Using GIS-based property tax records as an alternative to traditional household listing in area samples. *Proceedings of the Section on Survey Research Methods, American Statistical Association.* 2004:3750–3757.

Kalton G. *Introduction to Survey Sampling.* Newbury Park, CA: Sage; 1983.

Kalton G, Flores-Cervantes I. Weighting methods. *Journal of Official Statistics* 2003;19(2):81–97.

Kish L. *Survey Sampling*. New York: Wiley; 1965.

Lessler JT, Kalsbeek WD. *Nonsampling Error in Surveys*. New York: Wiley; 1992.

Lohr SL. *Sampling: Design and Analysis.* Pacific Grove, CA: Duxbury Press; 1999.

Mosca L, Ferris A, Fabunmi R, Robertson RM. Tracking women's awareness of heart disease. *Circulation* 2004;109:573–579.

Moy E, Bartman BA. Physician race and care of minority and medically indigent patients. *Journal of the American Medical Association* 1995;273(19):1515–1520.

Oldendick RW, Bishop GF, Sorenson SB, Tuchfarber AJ. A comparison of the Kish and last birthday methods of respondent selection in telephone surveys. *Journal of Official Statistics* 1988;4(4):307–318.

Särndal CE, Swensson B, Wretman J. *Model Assisted Survey Sampling*. New York: Springer-Verlag; 1992.

Thompson SK. Adaptive cluster sampling. *Journal of the American Statistical Association* 1990;85(412):1050–1059.

Troldahl VC, Carter RE. Random selection of respondents within households in phone surveys. *Journal of Marketing Research* 1964;1:71–76.

Waksberg J. The effect of stratification with differential sampling rates on attributes of subsets of the population. *Proceedings of the Survey Research Methods Section, American Statistical Association.* 1973:429–434.

Waksberg J, Levine D, Marker D. *Assessment of Major Federal Data Sets for Analyses of Hispanic and Asian or Pacific Islander Subgroups and Native Americans: Extending the Utility of Federal Data Bases.* Washington, DC: U.S. Department of Health and Human Services, Office of the Assistant Secretary for Planning and Evaluation; 2000. Available at http://aspe.hhs.gov/hsp/minority-db00/task2/index.htm.

Wolter KM. *Introduction to Variance Estimation.* New York: Springer-Verlag; 1985.

F.2.4 Analysis and Reporting

Americans for Nonsmokers' Rights (ANRF). *States and Municipalities with 100% Smokefree Laws in Workplaces, Restaurants, or Bars.* Available at http://www.no-smoke.org/pdf/100ordlist.pdf.

Brownson RC, Hopkins DP, Wakefield MA. Effects of smoking restrictions in the workplace. *Annual Review of Public Health* 2002;23:333–348.

Clark PI, Gardiner PS, Djordjevic MV, Leischow SJ, Robinson RG. Menthol cigarettes: setting the research agenda. *Nicotine & Tobacco Research* 2004;6(Suppl. 1):S5–S9.

Fleiss JL, Levin B, Paik MC. *Statistical Methods for Rates and Proportions.* 3rd edition. New York: Wiley; 2003.

Giovino GA, Sidney S, Gfroerer JC, O'Malley PM, Allen JA, Richter PA, et al. Epidemiology of menthol cigarette use. *Nicotine & Tobacco Research* 2004;6(Suppl. 1):S67–S81.

Mowery PD, Farrelly MC, Haviland ML, Gable JM, Wells HE. Progression to established smoking among US youths. *American Journal of Public Health* 2004;94(2):331–337.

Nazaroff WW, Singer BC. Inhalation of hazardous air pollutants from environmental tobacco smoke in US residences. *Journal of Exposure Analysis and Environmental Epidemiology* 2004;14(Suppl. 1):S71–S77.

Pirkle JL, Flegal KM, Bernert JT, Brody DJ, Etzel RA, Maurer KR. Exposure of the US population to environmental tobacco smoke: the Third National Health and Nutrition Examination Survey, 1988 to 1991. *Journal of the American Medical Association* 1996;275(16):1233–1240.

Shopland DR, Anderson CM, Burns DM, Gerlach KK. Disparities in smoke-free workplace policies among food service workers. *Journal of Occupational and Environmental Medicine* 2004;46(4):347–356.

U.S. Census Bureau. *Current Population Survey, February, June, and November 2003: Tobacco Use Supplement Technical Documentation CPS-03* [CD-ROM]. Washington, DC: Marketing Services Office, Customer Services Center, U.S. Bureau of the Census; 2006. Available at http://riskfactor.cancer.gov/studies/tus-cps/index.html.

U.S. Department of Health and Human Services (USDHHS). *The Health Benefits of Smoking Cessation: A Report of the Surgeon General.* Rockville, MD: USDHHS, Centers for Disease Control and Prevention, Coordinating Center for Health Promotion, National Center for Chronic Disease Prevention and Health Promotion, Office on Smoking and Health; 1990. USDHHS Publication No. [CDC] YO-K-116.

U.S. Department of Health and Human Services (USDHHS). *Tobacco Use Among U.S. Racial/Ethnic Minority Groups—African Americans, American Indians and Alaska Natives, Asian Americans and Pacific Islanders, and Hispanics: A Report of the Surgeon General.* Atlanta, GA: USDHHS, Centers for Disease Control and Prevention, Coordinating Center for Health Promotion, National Center for Chronic Disease Prevention and Health Promotion, Office on Smoking and Health; 1998.

U.S. Department of Health and Human Services (USDHHS). *The Health Consequences of Involuntary Exposure to Tobacco Smoke: A Report of the Surgeon General.* Atlanta, GA: USDHHS, Centers for Disease Control and Prevention, Coordinating Center for Health Promotion, National Center for Chronic Disease Prevention and Health Promotion, Office on Smoking and Health; 2006.

F.2.5 Enhancing Response Rates

Albright V. Current methodological issues in telephone interviewing. Presentation to the annual meeting of Bay Area Survey Evaluators, Researchers, and Statisticians, University of California, Berkeley, September 2003.

Albright V, Bye L. Integrating priority populations into comprehensive surveillance and evaluation systems: California's LGBT Population Survey. Paper presented at the 2003 National Conference on Tobacco or Health Conference, Boston, MA, May 2003.

American Association of Public Opinion Research (AAPOR). *Resources for Researchers.* 2006. Available at http://www.aapor.org/resources.

U.S. Department of Health and Human Services (USDHHS). *Effective Tobacco Control in Hispanic/Latino Communities: A Synopsis of Key Findings and Recommendations.* Atlanta, GA: USDHHS, Centers for Disease Control and Prevention, Coordinating Center for Health Promotion, National Center for Chronic Disease Prevention and Health Promotion, Office on Smoking and Health; 2004.

F.3 Contacts

Centers for Disease Control and Prevention, National Center for Chronic Disease Prevention and Health Promotion, Office on Smoking and Health

Internet address: tobaccoinfo@cdc.gov
Phone: 1-800-CDC-INFO

APPENDIX A: ADVANCE LETTER TO POTENTIAL HOUSEHOLDS, TELEPHONE SURVEY (ENGLISH)

ADVANCE LETTER TO POTENTIAL HOUSEHOLDS, TELEPHONE SURVEY (ENGLISH)

[USE LEAD AGENCY LETTERHEAD.]

[DATE]

Dear Household Members:

Your household has been selected to participate in a telephone survey about knowledge, attitudes, and behaviors related to tobacco use. This survey has been approved by [NAME LEAD AGENCY AND OTHER LOCAL RESEARCH PARTNERS]. Your participation in this study is voluntary, and any information you provide will be maintained in a confidential manner. The results of the study will be very important in helping your community health services address serious health issues among Hispanic and Latino persons as a result of tobacco use. We will select one adult at random in your household to complete the survey. An interviewer will be calling your house in the next week. He or she will be able to tell you more about the survey, select a respondent in your household, and conduct the survey by telephone. Even if you choose not to participate, please take a few moments to speak with our interviewer when he or she calls you.

Thank you for your help in this matter.

APPENDIX B: ADVANCE LETTER TO POTENTIAL HOUSEHOLDS, TELEPHONE SURVEY (SPANISH)

ADVANCE LETTER TO POTENTIAL HOUSEHOLDS, TELEPHONE SURVEY (SPANISH)

[USE LEAD AGENCY LETTERHEAD.]

[DATE]

Estimados miembros del hogar:

Este hogar ha ido seleccionado para participar en una encuesta acerca del conocimiento, las actitudes y los comportamientos relacionados con el uso del tabaco. Esta encuesta ha sido aprobada por [NOMBRE DE LA AGENCIA PRINCIPAL Y DE LOS OTROS ASOCIADOS LOCALES PARA EL ESTUDIO]. Su participación en este estudio es voluntaria y toda la información que usted nos dé se mantendrá de manera confidencial. Los resultados del estudio serán muy importantes para ayudar a los servicios de salud de su comunidad a confrontar serios problemas de salud que son consecuencia del uso del tabaco entre las personas hispanas y latinas. Seleccionaremos al azar a un adulto en su hogar para que complete la encuesta. Un(a) entrevistador(a) le llamará por teléfono a su hogar en la próxima semana. El/la entrevistador(a) podrá darle más información acerca de la encuesta, escoger un participante en su hogar, y hacer la encuesta. Aún si usted decide no participar, por favor dedique unos minutos a hablar con nuestro(a) entrevistador(a) cuando él/ella vaya a su hogar.

Muchas gracias por su cooperación.

APPENDIX C: ADVANCE LETTER TO POTENTIAL HOUSEHOLDS, IN-PERSON SURVEY (ENGLISH)

ADVANCE LETTER TO POTENTIAL HOUSEHOLDS, IN-PERSON SURVEY (ENGLISH)

[USE LEAD AGENCY LETTERHEAD.]

[DATE]

Dear Household Members:

Your household has been selected to participate in a survey about knowledge, attitudes, and behaviors related to tobacco use. This survey has been approved by [NAME LEAD AGENCY AND OTHER LOCAL RESEARCH PARTNERS]. Your participation in this study is voluntary and any information you provide will be maintained in a confidential manner. The results of the study will be very important in helping your community health services address serious health issues among Hispanic and Latino persons as a result of tobacco use. We will select one adult at random in your household to complete the survey. He or she will receive a $15 gift card as compensation for the time spent on the interview. An interviewer will be dropping by your house in the next week. He or she will be able to tell you more about the survey, select a respondent in your household, and conduct the survey. Even if you choose not to participate, please take a few moments to speak with our interviewer when he or she comes to your house.

Thank you for your help in this matter.

APPENDIX D: ADVANCE LETTER TO POTENTIAL HOUSEHOLDS, IN-PERSON SURVEY (SPANISH)

ADVANCE LETTER TO POTENTIAL HOUSEHOLDS, IN-PERSON SURVEY (SPANISH)

[USE LEAD AGENCY LETTERHEAD.]

[DATE]

Estimados miembros del hogar:

Este hogar ha ido seleccionado para participar en una encuesta acerca del conocimiento, las actitudes y los comportamientos relacionados con el uso del tabaco. Esta encuesta ha sido aprobada por [NOMBRE DE LA AGENCIA PRINCIPAL Y DE LOS OTROS ASOCIADOS LOCALES PARA EL ESTUDIO]. Su participación en este estudio es voluntaria y toda la información que usted nos dé se mantendrá de manera confidencial. Los resultados del estudio serán muy importantes para ayudar a los servicios de salud de su comunidad a confrontar serios problemas de salud que son consecuencia del uso del tabaco entre las personas hispanas y latinas. Seleccionaremos al azar a un adulto en su hogar para que complete la encuesta. Él o ella recibirá una tarjeta de regalo por un valor de $15 dólares como compensación por el tiempo que nos concedió para la entrevista. Un(a) entrevistador(a) pasará por su hogar en la próxima semana. El/la entrevistador(a) podrá darle más información acerca de la encuesta, escoger un participante en su hogar, y hacer la encuesta. Aún si usted decide no participar, por favor dedique unos minutos a hablar con nuestro(a) entrevistador(a) cuando él/ella vaya a su hogar.

Muchas gracias por su cooperación.

APPENDIX E: INFORMED CONSENT FORM, IN-PERSON SURVEY (ENGLISH)

ADULT TOBACCO SURVEY INFORMED CONSENT FORM

Purpose and Benefits

The Texas State Health Department is conducting a survey. This survey is to learn about the knowledge, attitudes, and behaviors related to tobacco use. This survey is being done among Hispanic/Latino adults. It is sponsored by the Centers for Disease Control and Prevention. Your taking the survey will help us to identify tobacco use problems and needs in your own community. It will also help to improve services and programs aimed at preventing or decreasing tobacco use and its health effects.

Procedures

Yearly, we will recruit about 2,250 adults 18 years of age or older to take the survey. The interview will take about 30 minutes to complete. The interview will include general demographic questions. It will also include questions related to tobacco use.

Safeguarding Privacy

Any information you provide will be maintained in a secure manner. No one but the interviewer will know how you answered the questions. The interviewer has signed a pledge to keep all information about you secure. Your name will be removed from all records involved in the survey. A number will be assigned to the survey questionnaire instead. Only project staff will have access to the study data. We will not use your name when we report results of the survey. The data we collect from you will be combined with data from other adults in El Paso. The combined data will yield a profile of community smoking and health.

Risks and Benefits

There are no known risks to you as a person taking this survey. There are no known direct benefits to you. However, the overall impact for your community may be great because new data on tobacco use will help to address a crucial health problem. You will receive a $15 gift card to compensate you for your time.

Rights as a Volunteer

Your taking the Adult Tobacco Survey is your choice. If you feel uneasy with any of the questions, you can refuse to answer. You may also skip questions you do not want to answer. You can stop the interview at any time. If you decide not to take part or to stop the interview, you will not lose any services that you are otherwise receiving.

If you have any questions about this survey, you may call [FIELD SUPERVISOR]. You may also call the Project Coordinator, [NAME, TELEPHONE NUMBER].

If you have questions about your rights in taking this survey, you may call [NAME, TELEPHONE NUMBER].

Respondent Agreement

The Adult Tobacco Survey has been explained to me. I consent to participate. I have had a chance for my questions to be answered. I know that I may refuse to participate or to stop the interview at any time without any loss of health care benefits that I am otherwise receiving. I understand that if I have questions about this survey or my rights in taking it, or if I feel I have been injured in this study, I may contact [NAME, TELEPHONE NUMBER]. No funds have been set aside to compensate participants for injuries.

______________________________ ____________________
Respondent Signature Date

______________________________ ____________________
Interviewer Signature Date

Copies: ☐ Respondent ☐ Project Coordinator

APPENDIX F: INFORMED CONSENT FORM, IN-PERSON SURVEY (SPANISH)

FORMULARIO DE CONSENTIMIENTO INFORMADO PARA LA ENCUESTA DEL TABACO PARA ADULTOS

Propósitos y Beneficios

El Departamento de Salud del Estado de Texas está realizando una encuesta. Esta encuesta es para aprender el conocimiento, las actitudes y los comportamientos relacionados con el uso del tabaco. Esta encuesta se está haciendo entre adultos hispanos/latinos y está patrocinada por Los Centros para el Control y la Prevención de Enfermedades. Su participación en la encuesta nos ayudará a identificar los problemas del uso del tabaco y las necesidades en su propia comunidad. También ayudará a mejorar los servicios y programas destinados a prevenir o disminuir el uso del tabaco y sus efectos hacia la salud.

Procedimientos

Cada año, nosotros estaremos buscando a cerca de 2,250 adultos de 18 años de edad o más para que participen en la encuesta. La entrevista durará como 30 minutos en completarse. La entrevista incluirá preguntas demográficas generales. También incluirá preguntas relacionadas con el uso del tabaco.

Protegiendo su privacidad

Cualquier información que usted proporcione se mantendrá de una manera segura. Aparte del entrevistador, nadie más sabrá cómo contestó usted las preguntas. El entrevistador ha firmado un compromiso para mantener de manera segura toda la información acerca de usted. Su nombre será eliminado de todos los documentos asociados con la encuesta. En cambio, se asignará un número al cuestionario de la encuesta. Solamente los miembros del personal tendrán acceso a los datos del estudio. Nosotros no usaremos su nombre cuando informemos acerca de los resultados de la encuesta. La información que usted nos dé se combinará con la información de otros adultos en El Paso. Los datos combinados producirán una descripción sobre la salud y el fumar dentro de la comunidad.

Riesgos y beneficios

No se sabe de ningún riesgo que le pueda suceder a usted como persona participante en esta encuesta. No se sabe de ningún beneficio directo hacia usted. Sin embargo, el impacto general en su comunidad será significativo porque el tener nueva información sobre el uso de tabaco ayudará a tratar un importante problema de la salud. Usted recibirá una tarjeta de regalo por un valor de $15 dólares para compensarlo(a) por su tiempo.

Derechos como voluntario(a)

Su participación en la Encuesta del Consumo de Tabaco para Adultos depende de usted. Si se siente incómodo(a) con algunas de las preguntas, usted puede negarse a contestarlas. También puede pasar por alto cualquier pregunta que no quiera contestar. Usted puede parar la entrevista en cualquier momento. Si decide no participar o interrumpir la entrevista, no perderá ningún servicio al que ya tenga derecho.

Si tiene alguna pregunta acerca de esta encuesta, puede llamar a [FIELD SUPERVISOR]. También puede llamar al/a la Coordinador(a) del Proyecto, [NAME, TELEPHONE NUMBER].

Si tiene preguntas acerca de sus derechos como participante en la encuesta, puede llamar a [NAME, TELEPHONE NUMBER].

Acuerdo del participante

Me han explicado en qué consiste la Encuesta del Consumo de Tabaco para Adultos. Yo doy mi consentimiento para participar. He tenido la oportunidad de que respondan a mis preguntas. Entiendo que puedo negarme a participar o interrumpir la entrevista en cualquier momento sin riesgo de perder ningún beneficio de atención médica que ya estoy recibiendo. Entiendo que si tengo preguntas sobre esta encuesta o sobre mis derechos como participante, o si pienso que el participar en este estudio me ha causado alguna lesión, puedo llamar a [NAME, TELEPHONE NUMBER]. No hay fondos monetarios disponibles para compensar a los participantes debido a lesiones personales.

______________________________________ _______________________

Firma del participante Fecha

______________________________________ _______________________

Firma del/de la entrevistador(a) Fecha

Copias: ☐ Participante ☐ Coordinador(a) del Proyecto

APPENDIX G: INFORMED CONSENT TEXT, TELEPHONE SURVEY (ENGLISH)

INFORMED CONSENT TEXT, TELEPHONE SURVEY (ENGLISH)

[The following is read to each respondent before beginning the interview. The respondent must agree to continue the interview after the following is read to him or her.]

"The Texas State Health Department is conducting a survey. This survey is to learn about the knowledge, attitudes, and behaviors related to tobacco use. This survey is being done among Hispanic/Latino adults. It is sponsored by the Centers for Disease Control and Prevention. Your taking the survey will help us to identify tobacco use problems and needs in your own community. It will also help to improve services and programs aimed at preventing or decreasing tobacco use and its health effects.

"Yearly, we will recruit about 2,250 adults 18 years of age or older to take the survey. The interview will take about 30 minutes to complete. The interview will include general demographic questions. It will also include questions related to tobacco use.

"Any information you provide will be maintained in a secure manner. No one but the interviewer will know how you answered the questions. The interviewer has signed a pledge to keep all information about you secure. Your name will be removed from all records involved in the survey. A number will be assigned to the survey questionnaire instead. Only project staff will have access to the study data. We will not use your name when we report results of the survey. The data we collect from you will be combined with data from other adults in El Paso. The combined data will yield a profile of community smoking and health.

"There are no known risks to you as a person taking this survey. There are no known direct benefits to you. However, the overall impact for your community may be great because new data on tobacco use will help to address a crucial health problem.

"Your taking the Adult Tobacco Survey is your choice. If you feel uneasy with any of the questions, you can refuse to answer. You may also skip questions you do not want to answer. You can stop the interview at any time. If you decide not to take part or to stop the interview, you will not lose any services that you are otherwise receiving.

"If you have any questions about this survey, you may call [FIELD SUPERVISOR]. You may also call the Project Coordinator, [NAME, TELEPHONE NUMBER].

"If you have questions about your rights in taking the survey, you may call [NAME, TELEPHONE NUMBER]. You may also call if feel you have been injured in this study. No funds have been set aside to compensate participants for injuries."

APPENDIX H: INFORMED CONSENT TEXT, TELEPHONE SURVEY (SPANISH)

INFORMED CONSENT TEXT, TELEPHONE SURVEY (SPANISH)

[The following is read to each respondent before beginning the interview. The respondent must agree to continue the interview after the following is read to him or her.]

"El Departamento de Salud del Estado de Texas está realizando una encuesta. Esta encuesta es para aprender el conocimiento, las actitudes y los comportamientos relacionados con el uso del tabaco. Esta encuesta se está haciendo entre adultos hispanos/ latinos y está patrocinada por Los Centros para el Control y la Prevención de Enfermedades. Su participación en la encuesta nos ayudará a identificar los problemas del uso del tabaco y las necesidades en su propia comunidad. También ayudará a mejorar los servicios y programas destinados a prevenir o disminuir el uso del tabaco y sus efectos hacia la salud.

"Cada año, nosotros estaremos buscando a cerca de 2,250 adultos de 18 años de edad o más para que participen en la encuesta. La entrevista durará como 30 minutos en completarse. La entrevista incluirá preguntas demográficas generales. También incluirá preguntas relacionadas con el uso del tabaco.

"Cualquier información que usted proporcione se mantendrá de una manera segura. Aparte del entrevistador, nadie más sabrá cómo contestó usted las preguntas. El entrevistador ha firmado un compromiso para mantener de manera segura toda la información acerca de usted. Su nombre será eliminado de todos los documentos asociados con la encuesta. En cambio, se asignará un número al cuestionario de la encuesta. Solamente los miembros del personal tendrán acceso a los datos del estudio. Nosotros no usaremos su nombre cuando informemos acerca de los resultados de la encuesta. La información que usted nos dé se combinará con la información de otros adultos en El Paso. Los datos combinados producirán una descripción sobre la salud y el fumar dentro de la comunidad.

"No se sabe de ningún riesgo que le pueda suceder a usted como persona participante en esta encuesta. No se sabe de ningún beneficio directo hacia usted. Sin embargo, el impacto general en su comunidad será significativo porque el tener nueva información sobre el uso de tabaco ayudará a tratar un importante problema de la salud.

"Su participación en la Encuesta del Consumo de Tabaco para Adultos depende de usted. Si se siente incómodo(a) con algunas de las preguntas, usted puede negarse a contestarlas. También puede pasar por alto cualquier pregunta que no quiera contestar. Usted puede parar la entrevista en cualquier momento. Si decide no participar o interrumpir la entrevista, no perderá ningún servicio al que ya tenga derecho.

"Si tiene alguna pregunta acerca de esta encuesta, puede llamar a [FIELD SUPERVISOR]. También puede llamar al/a la Coordinador(a) del Proyecto, [NAME, TELEPHONE NUMBER].

"Si tiene preguntas acerca de sus derechos como participante en la encuesta, puede llamar a [NAME, TELEPHONE NUMBER]. Usted también puede llamar si piensa que el participar en este estudio le ha causado alguna lesión. No hay fondos monetarios disponibles para compensar a los participantes debido a lesiones personales."

www.ingramcontent.com/pod-product-compliance
Lightning Source LLC
Chambersburg PA
CBHW081840170526
45167CB00007B/2863

* 9 7 8 1 4 9 9 5 7 1 6 4 6 *